HIDDEN SPRING

A BUDDHIST WOMAN CONFRONTS CANCER

also by Sandy Boucher

Discovering Kwan Yin, Buddhist Goddess of Compassion

Opening the Lotus: A Woman's Guide to Buddhism

Turning the Wheel: American Women Creating the New Buddhism

Heartwomen: An Urban Feminist's Odyssey Home

The Notebooks of Leni Clare (stories)

Assaults and Rituals (stories)

HIDDEN SPRING

A Buddhist Woman Confronts Cancer

Sandy Boucher

WISDOM PUBLICATIONS • BOSTON

Wisdom Publications
199 Elm St.
Somerville, MA 02144

© 2000 Sandy Boucher

Library of Congress Cataloging-in-Publication Data
Boucher, Sandy.
Hidden Spring: a Buddhist woman confronts cancer / Sandy Boucher.
p. cm.
ISBN 0-86171-171-8 (alk. paper)
1. Boucher, Sandy. 2. Buddhist women—United States—Biography.
3. Colon (Anatomy)—Cancer—Patients—United States—Biography.
4. Spiritual life—Buddhism. I. Title.
BQ734.B67 2000
294.3'092—dc21   00-032066
[B]

ISBN 0-86171-171-8.

05 04 03 02 01
6 5 4 3 2

Cover design by Graciela Galup
Interior by Gopa Design
Cover photo © Lasse Karkkainen/Photonica

Poems on pages vi, 131, 192 taken from *Japanese Death Poems:
Written by Zen Monks and Haiku Poets on the Verge of Death,*
© 1986, Tuttle Publishing, Boston. Reprinted with permission.

Poem on page 187 taken from *Chiyo-ni: Woman Haiku Master,*
© 1998, Tuttle Publishing, Boston. Reprinted with permission.

Wisdom Publications' books are printed on acid-free paper
and meet the guidelines for the permanence and durability
of the Production Guidelines for Book Longevity
of the Council on Library Resources.

Printed in the United States of America

To the memory of Rick Fields,
fellow Buddhist chronicler
and cancer buddy

and to Sandra Butler
for her intelligence, courage,
and boundless heart

In the heart of the fire
lies a hidden spring
Giun

Table of Contents

Acknowledgments

FIRST AMONG THOSE I wish to thank are the people at Highland Hospital: the oncologists, particularly Dr. Cutting and Dr. Yee; the oncology nurses, Bill Shanks and Sally Walker, Gondica Strykers and Wanda Brenni; the excellent women who keep the place running, Mary Ann Roberts, Darlene Reed, and Aisha Whitehead; and Michael Coombs, who used to tend the desk. It is because these people do their jobs so well that I'm alive. And I should say here that the buildings at Highland have been radically upgraded since my first experiences there in 1995–1996, and that Oncology now has its own private, well-appointed suite of rooms.

It's impossible to list all the people who helped me through the surgery and many weeks of chemotherapy, but I want to name some of you. First among those who helped were Nancy Berson and the Wandering Menstruals (Jane Ariel, Sandra Butler, Marinell Eva, Marcia Freedman, Nan Fink Gefen, Arlene Shmaeff, and Linda Wilson). Jennifer Berezan I thank for her music, and for the other ways in which she offered me aid and love. Tillie Olsen, Annie Hershey, and Osha Hibbard gave the balm of their longtime strong friendship. The Charlotte Maxwell Clinic was my steady support in hard periods. A number of healers gave freely of their time and energy: Barbara Wilt, Michael Broffman, Vicki Noble, Meera Chaturvedi, Margaret Pavel, Carol Newhouse, Bea Heinze-Westley, and Diana Seagiver. Then there were those who brought food, cleaned our house, worked in our yard, drove me to appointments, sent me money, cards, gifts, encouragement, remedies, and love. I tried listing all of you, and wound up with two dense pages of names, and more coming to mind. So I have decided simply to say to you, because you know who you are and what you gave, that your generosity helped me to live through the difficult cancer time. I can't thank you enough.

I want to acknowledge Crystal Juelson's efforts on my behalf, and thank her for insisting that I include in this book some description of the dissolution of our relationship, that it may remind others that the unraveling of marriages and partnerships is not unusual under the stress of life-threatening illness, and that no one is to blame.

I thank Susan Griffin and Harold Brodkey for their modeling of how to write about illness.

Those who read the manuscript and helped me with its revision are Nan Fink Gefen, Judith McDaniel, Marcia Freedman, and Sandra Butler. I am grateful to them for the careful attention they gave to my work.

Jan Feldman led the cancer support group that provided so much encouragement. She did so in a warm, insightful, and compassionate manner, for which I thank her with all my heart. Cheryl Jones has stood by me during the months of the writing of this book, helping me accept the grieving that inevitably arose. I am grateful to her for her skill and kindness.

The people at Wisdom Publications have been unfailingly enthusiastic about this book, and have labored to see that it goes out into the world in an appropriate and useful way. I can only hope that it lives up to their belief in it.

In the text itself and in the quotes before the chapters, I have acknowledged the wisdom of my many Buddhist teachers, but here I thank them again for guiding me, encouraging me, and facing me always toward the authenticity of my experience.

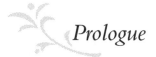 *Prologue*

It is the nature of all things that take form to dissolve again.

the Buddha

IN OCTOBER 1995 I went to a hospital in Oakland, where I live, for the medical test known as a sigmoidoscopy. Although I had been experiencing symptoms, I did not for a moment anticipate that there could be a serious problem. I expected to be told that I had some minor, easily corrected condition. But the test, instead, opened the door into the world of hospitals, surgery, and chemotherapy. The sigmoidoscopy showed a large tumor in my colon; a later colonoscopy confirmed it to be malignant. In a week I was having major surgery, and a month later began a course of chemotherapy that was supposed to last forty-eight weeks. My work, my intimate relationship, my home, my relations with friends, my body— every element of my life seemed sucked up into a dizzying vortex.

The one still point in this turning world was the Buddhist practice I had been cultivating for fifteen years. The formal meditation practice— all those hours of sitting still while emotions raged in me and my body clamored for relief—served me well. I had learned to be there for it all: to attend to my sensations, recognizing in that moment, as painful or imperfect or frustrating as it was, that this was the actual texture and content of my life; and then, because I noticed that nothing ever stayed the same, to experience its changing, and to know these thoughts, emotions, and sensations as the incessant flow of phenomena. This practice had steadied me through major crises in my life, providing a reliable base point to which to return, no matter what else was going on. During those years I had also been cultivating an attitude of spaciousness, acceptance, and compassion for others as well as myself. This training and its attendant cast of mind served me in the most trying times of my encounter with cancer, and also sometimes deserted me. My years of work with a unique and powerful teacher gave me some tools to meet the requirements of the illness and its treatment, when I could, and the compassion to be patient with myself and begin again, when I couldn't. I have tried to reveal how I applied the practice and benefited from the Buddhist perspective in many of the most difficult situations, hoping that my experience may be of use to the next person who opens that door.

My entry into the rich, sustaining tradition of Buddhism occurred in 1980 when I began to sit on a pillow and meditate. For the first three years, I thought I would just learn how to do the meditation, and have nothing to do with the furnishings of the religion out of which it came. Even so, because I am a curious person and like to orient myself in new activities, I began to study the texts of Buddhism, listen to what teachers said, and learn about the Asian roots of Buddhism; as I understood more, I began turning to Buddhist principles to shed light on my own experience. In a difficult situation, I would recall my reading or the insights I had gained in meditation, and ask myself what would be the action that would best promote the welfare of all concerned.

Over the fifteen years' time since I first sat down on a pillow and tried to pay attention, I have been doing meditation more or less faithfully both by myself and in groups, and with my principal teacher Ruth Denison in her center in the Mojave Desert of California. Ruth is one of the first generation of Western women who brought Buddhist practice to us in the United States; she had studied and meditated in Burma with a noted Theravada Buddhist teacher, who asked her to return here to teach. I myself went to Asia, where I lived for a short time as a Buddhist nun in Sri Lanka, and stayed in monasteries in Thailand and Burma. As part of my life as a writer and teacher I regularly study the texts of Buddhism, and continue meditating.

Most of all I have tried to apply the Buddhist principles in my daily life. That morning in the G.I. (Gastro-Intestinal) Laboratory at Summit Hospital gave me an opportunity to do so. I remember the doctor, a tall African-American man, talking to me after the test was completed. "When the growth is that big, we're ninety percent certain it's cancer. I'm calling your doctor right now. We want you in the hospital for major surgery in a week."

I am not a very spiritually adept person. Mostly I plod along, failing often, succeeding sometimes in my efforts at concentration and right action. But my years of practice and study had given me an understanding of life's task. When I received the news of cancer, I understood, Oh, yes, what is required of me now is that I be fully present to each new experience as it comes and that I engage with it as completely as I can. I don't mean that I said this to myself. Nothing so conscious as that. I mean that my whole being turned, and looked, and moved toward the experience.

Driving home from the hospital where the test had been performed, I remembered how, months before, my partner Crystal had urged me to get the sigmoidoscopy. For the period of her life just before I met her, in an extended detour from her career in music, Crystal had worked caring for the elderly. She remembered vividly one of her clients, an old woman dying of colon cancer because she had ignored the symptom of blood in her stool until it was too late. Now it was I who told Crystal that I had seen blood in my stool. "Please," she begged, "go get a sigmoidoscopy." But I was too busy writing, teaching my classes, and preparing to go to China to attend the United Nations Fourth World Conference on Women; I was spending time with the Wandering Menstruals, my support group of women over fifty, and my many other friends. I exercised regularly at a gym, and Crystal and I went out each weekend to hike or bike. I was living a busy, energetic existence, and I felt fine.

To Crystal's suggestions, I had snapped that I was not a seventy-year-old matron like her former client, and there was no time for a diagnostic test until I came back from China at the end of August. Now, driving home from Summit Hospital, I remembered her anxious face as she had listened to me. She mumbled that she hoped I was not making a mistake, and after that did not mention the sigmoidoscopy again.

What she feared had come to pass.

As I drove, I was just beginning to take in what had happened. In a crisis, we have many choices of how to react. We can reject the experience hysterically; we can rage against the injustice of it; we can go into deep denial and pretend it's not happening; we can move into the future, imagining a horrific outcome; we can retreat into obsessive worry, or sink into depression; and there are other possibilities. But after all those years of sitting still, cultivating awareness of the present moment, and perhaps also because I am by nature a rather positive person, I had none of those options. It seemed there was nothing to do but to be here fully for what would happen.

But this did not protect me from the usual thoughts and feelings, particularly in the initial shock. I remembered, later, a friend telling of hearing her own cancer diagnosis. "I thought I was on the mezzanine," she said, "and suddenly I was in the basement." It was like that.

Returning from the test, with the doctor's words echoing in my head, I walked up the back steps to my house. "Well, I'm fifty-nine years old," I thought. "I've published four books, I've experienced marriage and many intensely engaging love affairs, I've done honest political work, and I've traveled. I've lived my life as fully as I could. If this is the end, that will be all right."

Then I walked in the door, through the kitchen and into the living room, where Crystal was lying on the couch. She had been up most of the night working on a music project; I had seen her sleeping there when I left an hour or two earlier. Now she sat up and looked at me, her face creasing with concern. "What is it?" she asked. I walked across to the couch, knelt on the rug and burst into tears. Crystal put her arms around me as I choked out the news. And then she too was crying, as both of us felt the sadness of the coming ordeal, and the terror that my life might end.

Buddhist practice does not prevent anything, it does not shield us from anything. It softens and opens us to meet everything that comes to us.

PART ONE

1

Entering the System

Whatever comes, good or bad, don't make a move to avoid it.
Maurine Stuart Roshi

LIKE MOST AMERICAN BUDDHISTS who did not grow up in Asia or in Asian-American homes, I came to Buddhism as an adult. My mother was a Methodist. She had been raised in a religiously observant family, and declared that she had had enough of churchgoing in her life. However, she would always dress up herself, my brother, my sister, and me to go to Christmas Eve and Easter services at one of the Methodist churches in Columbus, Ohio, where we lived. It was my grandfather who took my sister and me to Sunday worship services (my brother, older than we, refused to go). The suffering Jesus on the cross in the great shadowy sanctuary fascinated me, for I had never seen a man so vulnerable. In Sunday school, when we read the story of the Good Samaritan, I was powerfully struck. I visualized the Samaritan getting down off his donkey to tend to the wounds of the man who had been robbed and beaten, and imagined him putting the wounded man up on his donkey to take him to an inn and care for him. I wanted to be like the Good Samaritan. But I never became seriously religious. By the time I was old enough to go to church by myself, I usually skipped the services and went instead to the Sunday-evening Methodist Youth Fellowship meetings, where we teenagers talked and ate, and sometimes danced or played games.

Halfway through high school I decided it was much more cool to be an agnostic like my father, and so I gave up church and youth fellowship for more racy pursuits. I became adept at telling off-color jokes, began to smoke cigarettes, and learned to drink beer. Yet I always circled in fascination around spirituality and religion. In the "Bible as Literature" course I took at college, I was stirred by the great primal stories of wars and betrayals, revelations, filial love, and sacrifice. Then during the sixties, as a married woman, I studied metaphysical books like the works of Vivikenanda, the founder of the Hindu sect of Vedanta, and his teacher Ramakrishna, and I began to understand that one could cultivate an expanded consciousness. I taught myself to do yoga postures from a book by an Indian yogi, and read esoteric texts like Eliphas Levi's *Transcendental Wisdom*, pondering their significance for my life.

But if I had a *practice,* it was that of writing. This was the one thread that sustained me through all the adventures and relationships that followed college. I was the first person in my immediate family to earn a university degree (from Ohio State University, chosen so that I could live at home and economize on expenses). I had begun writing stories and articles before high school, and by the time I was in my late teens, they were published now and then. The practice of writing—like meditation in its silence and solitude—became a necessity for me so that when I started meditating, that activity had a familiar feel to it. I was used to sitting silently for hours at a time, I was used to going inward, albeit with a different goal. Even during my most political period when, having left my husband and moved into a women's liberation collective in San Francisco, I gave heart and soul to the feminist activism of the seventies, I still found time to write. That inner exploration was the only quiet spot in a very outward-directed life.

When I first began to do a Buddhist practice, I used my daily morning meditation session to empty my mind to prepare me for the writing I would do that day. It was only later that I realized my spiritual practice had assumed an importance equal to writing in my life; then, I would pursue it not as a support for something else but for itself.

One of my ways of learning about the Buddhist path had been to study. So when the cancer came, I sought out the words of Buddhist teachers, women I had interviewed for my own books, whom I had sat with and watched develop over the years. They reminded me that always, whatever is happening, the task is to be fully present. I was drawn to the accounts of people facing serious illness and death, particularly fascinated by a group of Japanese death poems, and the poetry of the female haiku master Chiyo-ni. All of these writings emphasized the Buddhist truth of the continual change and flow of phenomena, in which dissolution and extinction occur as natural events in the cycle. Now I would have a closer relationship with this truth.

I entered the medical system, going for my first appointment in the surgery clinic at Highland Hospital. Highland is the county facility where the poor people of East Oakland go for their care, and where interns and residents from nearby medical schools train. Seen from the freeway, it juts up above the modest roofs of small stucco and frame houses—a great gray slab with its name in red neon across its curved front. If you should be unfortunate enough to be involved in a crash on that freeway, you will be lucky to be taken to Highland's trauma care facility, the best in the area. If you have no health insurance, Highland will treat you in its emergency room and clinics. Like forty-three million other Americans, I did not have health coverage, and so that morning Crystal and I drove out the freeway to that great gray edifice, and entered its crowded hallways.

I had been told I would be seeing Dr. Bold. What a name for a surgeon—shades of a wild-haired Mel Gibson character, jaw knotting as he sharpens his scalpel! I didn't know whether to feel amused or anxious.

We waited for several hours to see him, starting downstairs in the clinic lobby. If "lobby" suggests carpeting, cheerful pictures on the walls above comfortable chairs, and soft music piped in, your imagination is in the wrong hospital. At Highland, the floor was covered with worn, colorless linoleum and the walls were blank except for official-looking notices in Spanish, Chinese, Vietnamese, and Cambodian, telling the patients they should request a translator, who would be swiftly provided. A grainy TV set hanging from the ceiling blared talk shows. Crystal and I and the other patients, friends, and family sat in rows of straight plastic chairs, gazing in a sort of stupor at the bulletproof windows behind which a woman in a bright patterned head wrap and a man as intent and quizzical-looking as Spike Lee struggled to keep up with the stacks of clinic cards we had slipped, one by one, into Plexiglas containers on the counter.

After I had been checked in by the woman and handed my papers, Crystal and I took the elevator up to the third-floor surgery clinic. There we found a corridor with five-foot-high wooden partitions on either side. Inside the partitions, we sat on plastic chairs and looked at closed doors about four feet in front of us. At infrequent intervals a voice shouted names from the desk at the end of the corridor: "Jorge Velasco to room 3!" Then a worried-looking man, trailed by his plump, anxious wife and two small black-eyed children, made his way slowly down the row, stepping over feet, knees, canes, purses, baby carriages, crutches, grocery bags, tipped-over soda cans, and crumpled potato-chip bags. Someone might growl at him on the way; the rest of us gazed wistfully at him, wishing it were we who had been called. He fumbled to open the door with the wooden "3" stuck on it and disappeared inside, followed by his entourage. As the door closed, we who were left outside sank down once again into our slouched, subservient attitudes. It was as if a wind had blown across a stand of grass, lifting us, agitating us briefly, and then leaving us to sag into lethargy.

Here in the surgery clinic, I sat with Crystal at my side and thought of the small coiled monster in my intestine. Why would it be my *gut*? Why not my breast, like other women I knew? It was true that back home in Ohio, we fried our meat and potatoes and put salt even on raw apples, a habit I still had. And I liked to drink beer. But I hadn't smoked a cigarette in twenty years or eaten a steak in a long, long time, and I usually steamed my vegetables and tofu. So why did my colon invite in this grotesque little fellow traveler?

I stopped myself. The task now was to stay here, be fully present for this experience. As I had learned to do in my meditation practice, I tuned in to the sensations in my body. Legs and torso tense, hands gripped in my lap: my body was saying, Get me out of here! My feet shifted restlessly under my chair, wanting to be up and running. Buddhist practice asks us to be present for whatever we are experiencing even if it is painful or frightening, to pierce into the sensations, become fully attentive to them, and stay with them, being faithful to the actual reality of our lives. The goal is to achieve awareness of the subtle interaction of all elements of existence and experience the unending flow of phenomena without beginning or end. When we are able to do that, often it is possible to feel more expansive and accepting of our situation.

Focusing inward, I thought I might actually be able to have a perception of the tumor itself. But I felt nothing unusual in my lower belly. I had read about how the dancer Anna Halprin discovered her own colon cancer. While making a drawing of her body, she found herself coloring in a large black clump in her abdomen. How right it seemed that a dancer, after years of attention to her physical being, could sense the presence of something foreign, something dangerous. She went for a test the next day, and was diagnosed with advanced colon cancer.

Normally, through my meditation practice, I was in close communication with my body, but now I realized how little awareness I had focused on my physical being in the preceding months. Caught up with the preparations for China and the actual, arduous trip, I had been looking outward for the most part. Was my body rebelling against this neglect?

But in my years of spiritual practice I had come to understand one redeeming and heart-lifting truth: that we can always begin again. So we leave behind failure, neglect, inadequacy, resistance—we let them go, step into the present moment, and begin again. The Buddha's path is the Middle Way, balanced between harsh ascetic practice at one extreme, and uncontrolled sensual indulgence at the other. The Buddha himself tried the body-denying ascetic practices then current in ancient India, starving himself almost to death in the process, but came to understand that the body is our vehicle and must be nourished and cared for. So Buddhist practice is not about forcing anything, or judging oneself harshly when one is not able to maintain attention. We are urged to simply bring the mind back, without criticism or violence against ourselves. As Ruth Denison would put it, "Gently return." Gently return to yourself, to your own body/mind process as it expresses itself in this moment, and be with it. So I began again.

Sitting on the hard plastic chair, surrounded by the hustle and confusion, the stale air, and atmosphere of frustration and helplessness, with Crystal beside me making notes on her music score, I began to pay attention to my breath. As I had learned to do in my meditation practice, I felt the touch of the air on my upper lip and experienced the subtle expansion of my nostrils as the breath entered; I felt the breath's passage in my head and throat on its way to my lungs, and the slow release of the exhalation. Gradually I settled into this activity and surrendered to it, and soon I began to feel a difference in my body. The tightened muscles of my thighs softened a bit, my torso relaxed slightly against the back of my chair. I remembered the formula of one of the teachers I admired: "Breathing in I calm body and mind, breathing out I smile. This is the only moment; there is no other."

When we finally got in to see Dr. Bold, he turned out to be a neatly dressed young white man (but not as young, thank the goddess, as some of the residents we had seen bustling about in their new white coats, who looked like children playing doctor). We sat in a small, curtained cubicle open at the end to a counter piled chaotically with file folders, phones, instruments, vials of fluid, and boxes of gauze pads. As Dr. Bold talked to us, we heard voices from the other cubicles: "Does your father understand me when I talk to him, Mr. Tranh…?" "Now, Mrs. Jackson, your X-rays didn't turn out quite the way we'd hoped…." I found myself drawn in to the drama behind these remarks, mentally leaning toward the adjoining cubicle.

I was happy to see that Dr. Bold seemed able to shut out the voices around us. With an expression of concentration and concern, he got right to the point. "I've seen your sigmoidoscopy report. We'll want you to have a colonoscopy tomorrow morning, so we can go all the way up and check out your small intestine too, and I'll take a biopsy of the tumor while they're doing the colonoscopy, just to see whether it's malignant or not. But I should tell you that we are pretty certain that it is cancer."

Suddenly my breath stopped. As surely as if I had heard a bear ripping open my pack in the dead of night in the high Sierras (an experience I've actually had more than once), my body contracted like a fist and everything tingled. My mind seemed to lift up slightly from the top of my head and hover there.

"Then on Thursday we'll admit you and do the surgery," Dr. Bold continued.

Apologizing for his lack of artistic skill, he pulled a piece of paper from a stack and started to draw a picture of a wobbly tube, supposed to represent my colon. He drew straight lines across the tube to indicate the portion in which my nasty little troll had set up residence; they would remove a foot-long section of my bowel, he said, and sew the severed parts back together. Depending on what they found, I might or might not have to have a colostomy, a procedure that would leave me with a bag attached to my side, into which waste matter would empty.

I stared at Dr. Bold's drawing, seeing it shimmer with an unnatural clarity. His words marched by outside my mind as I tried to catch them.

"When we're in there, we'll see whether the tumor has eaten through the wall of the colon. If so, we'll take out some lymph nodes and send them to Pathology to see if they contain cancer cells."

I shifted my gaze from Dr. Bold's drawing to his clothes. I could not possibly respond to what he was saying: while we're *in there!!* lymph nodes! cancer cells! Dr. Bold was wearing a most unusual tie. From it the faces of jungle animals looked out at me. I peered into the round, strangely benign eyes of a lion as the doctor talked about the possibility of chemotherapy and/or radiation, depending on the results of the pathology investigation.

"Great tie," I said. "Where'd you get it?"

He blinked and glanced down at his chest. "Oh…the World Wildlife Fund, I guess…."

I smiled and nodded, happy to learn that he was an animal lover. Didn't that bode well for me?

Then I caught myself. Okay, Sandy, come back here! I heard the voice of a beloved Zen master, Maurine Stuart Roshi, urging me, whatever was going on, to stay right here and meet it. At a conference on women and Buddhism, Maurine had stood before a roomful of women and challenged us, "Whatever comes, good or bad, don't make a *move* to avoid it!" Her voice boomed out with a great temple bell's deep resonance. Shivers had run up my back as I received this injunction; it was as if the heart of Buddhism were expressed in this one phrase. Stand fully in the stream of your life, meet each event with all you have; don't step aside or sneak away, or try to creep out the back door. Stop denying and quibbling. Truly honor your own precious being and enter the endless complexity of what is offered to you in this moment. Remembering Maurine's words, I struggled to return to the present with my mind and body to receive the information Dr. Bold was giving me. *Don't make a move to avoid this.*

Leaning forward, I concentrated hard on Dr. Bold's description of the four stages of colon cancer. Stage one: completely contained. You're home free. Stage two: it's eaten through the wall but has not gone to the lymph nodes. Still pretty good. Stage three: Through the wall and into the lymph nodes. Here we have a big problem, since cancer cells may have escaped the lymph nodes to wander somewhere else in the body. Stage four: You're full of cancer and you might as well take a trip to the Bahamas in the few months left to you. When they opened me up, Dr. Bold explained, they might find any one of these situations.

"Do you have any questions?"

He was looking at his watch. Once again I was aware of the voices from behind the curtains. They spoke of treatment options, described surgical procedures. I realized that they were almost all doctors' voices; the patients were passive and grateful just to be seen, and sometimes not understanding what was being said. At Highland, things happened so slowly and then so fast. I had waited three hours, and I had spent roughly seven minutes with a doctor I'd never seen before. There were pressing things he had to communicate to me, all the while, I presume, feeling the urgency of all those others waiting in the narrow corridor outside.

I searched for a question and, grasping at my work to give me a sense of continuity, asked when I would be able to return to teaching my classes.

Dr. Bold looked up from writing in the chart. "This is *major surgery*," he said. "Give yourself *at least* a month to recover."

As we rode the elevator down to the pharmacy, Crystal took my arm. Her touch was warm and light, and I was glad for the contact.

The pharmacy was a long room with chairs lining one side and two counters at the other; up high, numbers flashed on a board. Crystal and I sat down on some empty chairs. Here in the pharmacy, the shortest wait was an hour and a half, and since everyone had already waited so long to see their doctors, I could feel the frustration of the thirty or forty people there. It seemed that to comfort themselves, everyone had been eating snacks, and dropping their trash on the floor. Toddlers lurched through sticky puddles of soda; discarded chip bags and sandwich wrappers rustled below the row of seats. A potbellied white man in a studded belt, big motorcycle boots and a black T-shirt with "Hells Angels" written across the back ran his hand through his wiry shoulder-length gray hair and squinted at us. An African-American man with big bronze muscles and a clunky white cast on his foot began to yell at the Asian clerk, "I been here for an hour, and I want my painkiller!" The clerk met his fury with an impassive face and asked him what his number was. A round-headed, brightly dressed woman, tiny as a child—perhaps Hmong, from Cambodia—squatted against the wall. Nobody read anything. They talked, moaned, shouted, laughed, complained, argued; and one young African-American woman wept quietly, looking ashamed of her tears.

This, I thought, was "Mother Highland." I had heard the hospital described that way by Maylie Scott, a Zen priest and former psychiatric social worker. "It's so crucial that it be out there in East Oakland," Maylie had told me. "There are people whose only access to care is there. They're born at Highland; when they have accidents or fights they're taken to its emergency room; their babies are born there; if they go crazy they wind up in the psych ward; when they're sick they go to the clinics; and when the end comes they die there. Highland is like a mother to this whole population." And to me as well, I thought. Thank the universe that Highland exists.

Between long silences, Crystal and I muttered to each other about logistics. Who would drive me to the hospital for the colonoscopy tomorrow. Whom to call.

And I breathed, remembering Maurine Stuart Roshi's commanding presence.

Finally my number flashed on the board and I got up to go to the thick Plexiglas window. With the amount of drugs back there, it made sense that the pharmacists were shielded by bullet-proof glass. Under my arm as we walked out was the "GoLightly" that would clean out my intestine tonight to provide the surgeons with a clear view tomorrow.

"Not really a fun day, was it?" I said to Crystal.

She glanced at me, and I caught a glimpse of her terror. For that instant she looked like a small, scared person, utterly vulnerable, and my heart opened to her. Then the moment was gone. She shook her head, agreeing, and I saw the lift of her chin as she turned away.

2

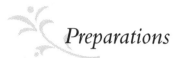

Preparations

*If we totally experience hopelessness, giving up all hope of
alternatives to the present moment, we can have a joyful
relationship with our lives, an honest, direct relationship, one
that no longer ignores the reality of impermanence and death.*

Pema Chodron

CRYSTAL AND I HAD MET at an artists' retreat at Vallecitos, New Mexico,
near Taos, four years before. She had been the first person I saw as I drove
up to the big old farmhouse set in a meadow next to a stream. In answer
to my question, she leaned back from arranging something in a VW
camping van and told me, yes, this was the place. A slender woman somewhere near my age, she regarded me from bright blue eyes beneath a
mane of thick blond-gray hair brushed back from her forehead. Tired
from the journey and annoyed by the rutted road leading to the house,
I simply thanked her for the information, and parked my car. That
evening at dinner, I learned her name and that she had come here to
compose music. In the following days, I settled in to work on a novel.
Meeting in the kitchen of the house, where all the residents ate their
meals, Crystal and I talked about music and writing, about the beauty of
the mountainous countryside around us, about Crystal's planned trip to
India. Each of us had recently left a relationship and had no intention of
starting another. In the yard, eating lunch in the dappled shade of a cot-
tonwood tree, we talked about our respective plans to live alone for a few
years before opening ourselves to another love relationship.

Soon we began to drive out into the countryside in Crystal's van to visit
the little towns and the ancient sites of the cliff dwellers. On those days
of driving and hiking I learned of Crystal's strong appreciation of nature

and sense of adventure, and I felt her gentleness. She told me of her deep but ambivalent engagement with music. She was the daughter of a pianist mother who had given up her concert career to raise Crystal in her small Washington hometown. Crystal had been an only child, often left alone while her mother taught piano lessons many hours a day to support them. Her mother had been strict and demanding where music was concerned, not nurturing Crystal's confidence in her own natural talent. Still, Crystal pursued music, and after leaving her marriage, while raising her own daughter in Santa Barbara, she had done almost all the work required to earn a Ph.D. in composition. But she was unable to continue the program, giving up her music to work as an elder-care aide. At the same time, she learned to be a masseuse. Now, aided by an inheritance after her mother's death, with her daughter away at college, Crystal was determined to return to composing New Music while supporting herself as a masseuse. (She explained to me that New Music was the term for contemporary classical music.) I was impressed with her talent and her courage.

Crystal asked about my lifestyle, in which I worked independently, earning a living teaching writing workshops and doing private writing consultation in the Berkeley/Oakland area. I learned that while she had only some slight knowledge of Buddhism, she was open to spiritual practice and had meditated in various ways. Close in age (she a few years younger), committed to our work, and happy in the out-of-doors, we became friends. And then, despite both of our intentions to postpone involvement, we began to feel strongly attracted to each other. Under the vast blue New Mexico skies, in the idyllic environment of the artist colony, we became lovers. Our intimacy awakened great happiness and hope in me, even though initially I struggled with it, wanting to honor my decision to stay single for a while. Then one day, standing in the meadow before the old house, looking down the hill to the sun-splashed trees lining the stream, I felt a certainty that Crystal was my true partner, the person with whom I was to spend the rest of my life. This was a revelation as unexpected as my earlier sudden awareness that my spiritual practice had become as important to me as my writing. In response, Crystal opened to me, and we began a passionate relationship.

A few months later, we set off for Asia together, and when we returned Crystal moved from her former home in Santa Barbara to live with me in Oakland.

Now, four years later, she drove me to the hospital where I would undergo the colonoscopy, and sat with me a few days later to learn that the growth in my colon was as nasty as it had looked: it was a malignant tumor.

The Buddha's First Noble Truth, known as *dukkha* (in Pali, the language of the original Buddhist canon), is that we suffer. Apprehension of this truth had been a foundation of my training with my Buddhist teacher Ruth Denison. In those sessions at Dhamma Dena, her center in the Mojave Desert, *dukkha* was kept always in the forefront of our minds, until I understood that simply to inhabit a human body is to experience discomfort, dis-ease, dissatisfaction, pain both physical and mental. The Buddha's First Noble Truth lets us know that suffering is not an aberration from some mythic state of constant happiness reminiscent of a beer ad or a shampoo commercial, with the wind perpetually ruffling our hair: suffering is simply a condition of life.

We experienced *dukkha* in varying degrees as we sat in meditation, as we performed the movement practice that Ruth Denison is known for, and as we worked in the stark desert environment of her meditation center; we examined the many textures and intensities of suffering in our own bodies and minds. Instead of running away from it, denying it, or stoically enduring it, we observed our suffering, practicing to allow it to exist with some equanimity. After, the acknowledgment of *dukkha* carried over into our daily lives.

With aging comes physical vulnerability; the body erupts now and then with painful difficulties. While I had thought of myself as a big, robustly healthy Midwesterner—and indeed had been that for most of the years of my life—menopause gave me some more nuanced perspectives on my physical existence. That passage had been rough for me, and included a loss of balance that led to two broken arms, one of them a complicated break that occasioned many months of physical pain and mental uncertainty. Then I fell off a bicycle and had to have an operation on my knee. Except for the first broken arm, which I was able to pay for, the second injury and the knee operation had to be dealt with at Highland Hospital. My many afternoons in the clinics at Highland drove home to me the omnipresence of suffering.

So when the cancer was diagnosed, I did not imagine that there was something wrong or terribly unfair in my having this disease. Others, like my acupuncturist Barbara, a Buddhist and dear friend, agreed. A small, compact woman who radiates intensity and concern, Barbara sat opposite me in her treatment room and fixed me with her brown eyes. "It's not really surprising," she said. "Our environment is full of toxins; cancer is an epidemic. Why *wouldn't* you have it?"

I saw her logic; this attitude made my task easier.

Of course I still often thought about the causes of cancer. Our air, our food, our water were laced with poisons; and nobody was doing very much about it—certainly not the so-called regulatory agencies. I had been reading newspaper reports of carcinogens in our gasoline, and how here in California toxic pesticide use had soared in the preceding five years; additionally, the stories pointed to pollution from the illegal manufacture of methamphetamines in some parts of California. How could this not affect my vulnerable, permeable human body?

Another possible cause was lifestyle. Did I consume too many hot dogs and French fries as an adolescent? Then there was heredity: was it my family's fault? And what about all that suppressed rage, grief, or other negative emotions churning in me with no way to get out except to create a disease? This explanation I rejected, not just because it did not ring true for me (though I do grant that for some people it may be helpful), but because it seemed to ask me to take on a false burden of responsibility that ignored both the larger landscape of causality and my need to deal with the crisis by being in the moment.

So I thought about all these possible causes, but I was instructed most by the classic Buddhist story of a man shot by an arrow. He's lying on the ground, seriously wounded. One person comes to help. She examines the arrow, and speculates on who may have made it and who might have shot it. She looks at the point of entry in the man's chest and calibrates the angle of approach and the possible speed with which the arrow traveled. All the while the man is dying. The other person who's come to help notices the victim's suffering and says, No, no, what is needed is not this inquiry, but to extract the arrow and treat the wound!

The story is a metaphor for Buddhist practice. It's why I disagree when people refer to Buddhism as a philosophy. Buddhism does have many philosophical dimensions to engage those interested in such matters, but it should never be understood solely in that way. It is, rather, a transformative process of liberation, a *method* designed to pull the arrows out of our chests and set us on the road to healing.

For me, the story strongly emphasized the need to stick to the demands of the moment. Yes, the network of causation for cancer did need to be addressed, and particularly the steady poisoning of our environment, but a patient preparing for major surgery and possibly a long siege of chemotherapy has other priorities. I had other priorities.

I had seen the growth in my colon. During the sigmoidoscopy the doctor in charge had invited me to look at the TV monitor. I watched as the miniature camera on the end of a flexible tube moved through my lower intestine, revealing a clean, shiny tunnel. Seeing this most private and hidden organ revealed, I felt like a voyeur. Then the camera went around a corner and practically bumped into something growing out from the wall of the tunnel. It looked like a clump of different kinds of tissue massed together, with blood vessels crawling over it. I glanced sideways at the doctor, seeing a fixed, grim expression on his handsome mahogany face. I looked back at this thing growing inside me. It was like a little monster, grotesquely wrapped around itself, ready to spring out and attack me. Yes, no question. There it was.

Later, as Dr. Bold talked to me, telling me that I was lucky I had come in now, for the tumor would soon have blocked my colon completely and with dire consequences, I was grateful that I had seen it. I had no doubts how I felt about its presence, size, or appearance. I would need no second opinion. I wanted it out of there.

In the few days before the surgery, Crystal went with me to appointments and sat in the crowded waiting rooms at Highland Hospital with her score on her lap, looking down at the notes that were like clusters of tiny grapes on a spidery arbor. She had been commissioned to write a choral work for a community chorus, and her deadline was near. In our lives together since Vallecitos, Crystal had focused on developing her massage practice and buying a house. This choral work was her return to music, and while she was thrilled at the opportunity, anxiety gripped her. She stayed up late to work on the score. She worried, doubted, and pushed herself beyond her strength. We were so opposite in our personalities: I would calmly measure my work habits, trusting that I would be able to accomplish what I set out to do.

While we waited, I sometimes watched her. Her hair was more gray now than when I had first met her. She was fifty-four years old. I had always loved the lines etched in the fine blond skin of her face, embarrassing her when I spoke of them, but now as I watched her I could see how much more deeply they had delineated themselves. The pressure of this composing job, combined with the crisis of my illness, was almost too much for her to contain. Crystal's nature was to expect the worst to happen, and she scrambled to avert future disaster. Because of our different perspectives, we often fought, our battles typically revolving around money. Early in our respective lives we had developed opposite accommodations to money. In response to a mother who counted pennies and gave reluctantly, I had made a decision to pay very little attention to money, to treat it casually. Reacting to her own family situation, Crystal had learned to focus with great care and particularity on money matters. So we often came into conflict, Crystal insisting that I pay attention to finances, and I refusing to put my time and energy there. In these battles we wounded and disappointed each other. The conflict surfaced again and again, but we did not really confront our differences and try to find a middle way and instead fell into a dangerous habit, which was to avoid the difficulties and go on as if all were well. Since those halcyon days in New Mexico, a distance had developed between us, a wariness of each other. Still, none of this could change the fact that I loved Crystal and believed that she would be my partner until I died.

Faced with the surgery, I canceled my classes and arranged to postpone the other responsibilities in my life. I had just signed a contract to write a book on Buddhism. I decided not to tell my editor in Boston that I had cancer and was about to be operated on; I had to trust that I would be able to begin the book after I recovered from the surgery.

And I wondered whom to tell. My parents and my brother were dead. With my older sister Wanda, who lives in Florida, I have a distant, amicable relationship. We had chosen very different paths: while I had finished college and left Columbus for New York City, Wanda had converted to Catholicism upon her marriage and given birth to six children. She had moved in next to my parents in a house my father built for her, and she and her husband raised their children there. Now, with the children grown and raising families of their own, Wanda lived in comfortable retirement with her husband. We communicated through greeting cards on holidays. She would not be among the first people I would call.

The first ones to know had to be the Wandering Menstruals, a group of women with whom I had been meeting monthly for the past six years to discuss menopause and aging. Among the eight of us, some were heterosexual and married, some lesbian; all the women except me were mothers. The Menstruals, along with several other friends, had become my family. Often in our meetings we had discussed how we would respond to a health crisis for one of our members. We had made a commitment to support each other through life's vicissitudes until we died, but our commitment had been mostly theoretical, up to now. My cancer presented us with our first emergency.

I hesitated before calling Sandra Butler, first among the Menstruals with whom I had a strong personal relationship. Five years earlier her partner had died of breast cancer; together they had written a book and had worked with others to found the Women's Cancer Resource Center. Later she herself had been operated on for thyroid cancer. Hadn't this been enough already? I steeled myself to hear her say, "I can't be part of this." Instead, after the first stunned silence, she asked, "How are you?" and then said, "We'll have to make a P.L.A.," Sandy's code for "plan of action." "Are you sure," I asked, "that you want to help with this? I'll understand completely if you say no." Sandy did not hesitate. "Absolutely, I do. I'm coming over!"

Fifteen minutes later she arrived at my door. She enveloped me in a huge hug. Sandy is six feet tall, just like me; when shorter people hug me, I have to bend down to meet them: when Sandy enfolds me we meet on the same satisfying level. Then she stepped back to give me a look that was piercing and compassionate at the same time.

"Let's sit down and talk this over," she said.

Sandy grew up in New York and has that East Coast confidence and deftness. She reads everything from the *New York Times* to studies on racism in America, from the latest feminist tome or literary novel by a woman to esoteric texts on Jewish spiritual practice, and has an opinion on most matters, which she freely shares. She had worked for years in the field of violence against women, having written one of the earliest books on that subject; she traveled to the Northwest, the Midwest, and as far as Alaska to give speeches and lead trainings for the volunteers who staffed battered women's centers.

Even in jeans and a sweatshirt, Sandy looked carefully dressed, brisk and efficient, her dark hair lying in waves across her high forehead and her eyes intent behind fashionable dark-rimmed glasses.

"All right, girl," she said. "First, you tell me everything." Reaching into her large black tote bag, she pulled out a legal pad and pen.

While I talked she listened, took notes, and shot questions at me. "So what *exactly* did they find?" "When do you go in for the surgery?" "Whom have you told?"

When I finished, she made some final notes and then leaned toward me.

"I'm going to call the other Menstruals and anyone else you'd like, and we'll decide how to organize things. Now you and I are going to make a list of the appointments you have and if Crystal can't go with you, one of us will take you and stay with you. And then we'll talk about any other needs you have and how we can meet them."

Fifteen minutes later, Sandy put her legal pad back into her bag and prepared to go. Then for a moment she sat looking at me. "I'm so sorry you have to go through this," she said.

Before she left she hugged me again, and I took comfort from her embrace, and from her capability. Sandy would rally the Wandering Menstruals, and they would act as the inner circle, communicating out with my larger community. I was glad to let more experienced others organize my care, particularly since I had no clear idea what I would need.

I had to announce to my students that I would be canceling some classes. These are writing classes for women that I teach independently. That night the "continuing" class was meeting in the living room that Crystal had so carefully decorated in shades of beige and rose. My students sat among the large beautiful ficus plant and palms that Crystal nurtured. Two years earlier, with her inheritance, she had made the down payment on this modest house, where I enjoyed teaching my classes.

When I told my students that I would be undergoing surgery in a few days, a woman spoke from the couch. "I'll stay all night in the hospital with you." I was confused, since I did not know her well. She was a divorced mother of four, a woman of intelligence and verve. Then someone else spoke up. "So will I," said this large, brown-haired woman in her soft Southern accent. She worked as a nurse in San Francisco, and gave the impression of great gentleness. I didn't know what to say. I had never been hospitalized before. Would it be appropriate for someone to stay all night with me? Would I need that kind of attention?

I called my political friends from the Graduate Theological Union. We were to give a presentation about our experience at the Beijing conference two days before my surgery. I decided to go ahead and participate.

On the telephone down to Joshua Tree in the Mojave Desert, I talked with Ruth Denison and the people who live there with her. Our conversations were factual, tentative; I would not know until after the surgery whether the cancer had invaded my lymph nodes. I spoke with my Buddhist friends in the Bay Area, who offered to come to the hospital and asked to be kept informed.

And I called Nancy Berson, a former writing student who had become a dear friend. Nancy had survived bladder cancer when she was in her early thirties, and now counseled people with cancer. "I won't come to see you in the hospital," she told me in her characteristically blunt way, "but if you'd like someone to coordinate the phone calls, I'm happy to do that." It was a great relief to turn the calls over to Nancy, for after speaking to the people closest to me, I had grown tired of telling the same story over and over again as more people in the community learned that I was in trouble and called to offer their help.

In the days before the surgery, when I was not busy with phone calls, I went often to walk in Mountain View Cemetery. The cemetery is an expanse of green opening amid the streets and traffic lights, shops and houses of my Oakland neighborhood. One enters through wide portals, circles around a fountain leaping high, and travels up an avenue bordered by great spreading oaks and magnolia trees with white creamy blossoms, like pale flames amid the dark leaves. On the higher reaches, the tombs of the titans of Oakland history stand next to each other on curving drives.

For years I had jogged in this graveyard, picnicked in it, walked in it. One morning while running on a high drive, I had glanced into the bushes on the slope to my left and stopped in wonderment. A group of little fox pups gazed up at me, startled, curious. They had been tumbling in among the shrubs, and they looked up in mid-action, one rollicking on top of another, one squatting to poop. The mother was nowhere to be seen. I stood and crooned to these creatures, and even thought I might be able to touch them. But as I approached, hand out, they scrambled away into the bushes, their small red-brown behinds disappearing among the weeds.

Another day I had watched a brown-feathered mother duck lead her five fluffy ducklings in a wobbly parade across the macadam from one pond to another. Under the trees, and up the slope among the graves, the stray cats sat watching, their eyes hooded, like gamblers bluffing until they could make their winning move. The next day when I came to jog in the early morning, I had found a duckling squashed flat on the pavement, the victim of a passing automobile's tire. Yet despite the dangers, each year the ducks mated, bore, and raised their ducklings here in the several ponds.

Now I sat on the grass of a high slope, under a huge spreading oak, and held a conversation with myself. Beneath a murky clouded sky, the tombs of the wealthy looked like bizarre little houses. They were built of pale stone or concrete, with polished marble columns and porticos, copper filigreed doors; caryatids stood in regal poses holding up the roof of one, marble angels bowed in grief at the door of another.

Down farther, where the humbler folk lay under the sod, I had just been walking among the gravestones, looking at the names—Chinese, Vietnamese, Hispanic, Jewish, Irish. On one new-looking stone, a photograph showed a young dark-skinned man with hair pulled back in a ponytail. His chin was lifted in defiance, his eyes challenging. Eighteen years old. Obviously much loved, because his people had left a pot of yellow chrysanthemums—real flowers, not the artificial blooms sprouting from other graves. I had just been listening to a radio program about young Hispanic kids who were gang members, and their short, violent lives. Perhaps he had been one of those bold ones. How terrible he had to die so young.

Sitting up here, I could hear a sprinkler thunking against its own spray and the distant murmur of freeway noise from down below. In this quiet, the trees moved just a little, their leaves shuddering in response to a breeze so gentle I could barely feel it. My belly hurt; ever since the colonoscopy there had been an ache there, probably from the "insult"—as my acupuncturist called it—of having that thing shoved up me.

Tears pressed at my eyes. I was sorry this was happening to me. I saw no meaning in it, no significance or lesson to be learned. But I knew I had no choice, just as so many other people have had no choice. I thought of my mother, remembering a time when she, normally a reticent woman, became uncharacteristically revealing as she told of the birth of my brother, her first child. The whole family had been sitting at the table after a holiday dinner. Her eyes bright with excitement, as if startled by her own loquacity, my mother told how for many hours she had endured contractions, and no baby came. At that time, in the late twenties, women waited out their labor in rocking chairs in the delivery room. So my mother sat and rocked all through the night, and her only comfort was the thought that in those same moments, all around the globe, a certain number of women like her sat rocking, enduring, waiting.

I was struck by my mother's story, for it spoke of surrender and of a larger empathy than I had known her to have. It expressed the Buddhist understanding of the interdependence of all beings. My mother had understood that she was not alone, that her experience was echoed in other women, and she was able to be nurturing to herself. Just so, the Buddhist principle that our lives are fundamentally joined with the lives of all other creatures is the source of compassion. To realize that we are the same in our suffering and joy, that we wish for the same things and fear the same things, is to awaken the desire in ourselves to act for the benefit of other beings. This compassion is a central value in Buddhism. It is embodied in the figure of the *bodhisattva*, who practices in order to achieve full enlightenment, but at the moment before achieving her or his goal, vows that she or he will not achieve full liberation until every being is enlightened. Then the bodhisattva turns back to the world and acts to alleviate suffering and awaken all beings to their true nature.

Bodhisattvas are not necessarily Buddhists. We have all known individuals in our daily life who respond with kindness and caring to everyone they meet. Perhaps the Good Samaritan was a bodhisattva. Zen priest Taigen Daniel Leighten has written a book called *Bodhisattva Archetypes*, in which he describes the classical bodhisattvas and then draws parallels with contemporary figures such as Daniel Elsberg and Mother Theresa, historical figures such as Francis of Assisi, whose actions sustain and enlighten others.

I had been strongly drawn to one celestial bodhisattva, the goddess Kwan Yin, for many years. Now as I sat in the graveyard, I felt myself impelled to pray to her. This surprised me, for I had been a skeptic on the subject of "goddesses." From my very political seventies' perspective, any deity was simply someone's fantasy-escape from reality. When my friends began, in the early eighties, to speak about the goddess-venerating cultures of antiquity and to seek to invoke the Great Goddess and other such figures, I swiftly rejected the ideas as irrelevant, distractions from the real work of making social change. When I began meditation practice, I found myself involved in Theravada Buddhism, the most ancient and austere of the several Buddhist traditions. In Theravada Buddhism, there are no gods; the Buddha himself was a human being. I found this refreshing, and was never really interested in the celestial beings venerated in some other forms of Buddhism.

Then, in 1982, a few years after I began Buddhist sitting, I was taken to an art museum in Kansas City, where I had gone on a book tour; there I encountered a life-sized wooden statue of Kwan Yin from twelfth- or thirteenth-century China. She sat gently smiling down at me, splendid, the Chinese bodhisattva of compassion, the most venerated goddess in all of Asia. Looking up at this exquisite figure, I felt all at once an astonishing spectrum of emotions, from intense sorrow all the way to quiet delight. Her meditating face expressed an equanimity that I found immensely comforting. From then on Kwan Yin was present in my life. My partner and I created a greeting card featuring her image and sold it. I read about her and collected pictures of her over the years. I noticed statues of her that presided over the Chinatown shops and restaurants I entered. I went to the City of Ten Thousand Buddhas in Talmage, California to see her enshrined among ten thousand small buddha images by Chinese monks and nuns. As I took more interest in women's spirituality, I found Kwan Yin entirely compatible with the pantheon of goddesses that women invoke. Over the years, as I learned more about Kwan Yin, I had to examine my formerly negative attitude to the feminine divine, and ask myself what a goddess actually *was* to me. I came to understand that a female deity represents a greater principle or truth, a source of wisdom, compassion, power; she provides a reminder of that larger reality and also evidence that the divine, the spiritual, the transcendent, can be visualized in a specifically female form. Whether that being exists in actuality as an energy in the world or a visible presence, I sometimes believe to be true and sometimes doubt.

What Kwan Yin most clearly embodies is the quality of compassion. She is called "She Who Hears the Cries of the World," and steps forward to help all suffering beings. Meditating on Kwan Yin—as she sits by the river holding a willow branch, or as she stands on a lotus blossom holding her vial containing the elixir of compassion to pour out over the world—can soften our hearts and open us to the truth that we share our lives with all beings, human and otherwise. She asks us to listen, as she does, to the cries of the world, and to begin always by giving compassionate care to ourselves.

Kwan Yin was particularly present to me in October 1995 because of my trip that previous summer to the Fourth World Conference on Women. Knowing I would be in China, the birthplace of Kwan Yin (or "Guan Shih Yin," as the Chinese call her), I made inquiries and found that there is an actual location in China where she is said to reside. So, with a Chinese-American friend who is a devotee of Kwan Yin, I made a pilgrimage to an island in the South China Sea called Putuo Shan, a place dedicated wholly to Kwan Yin. During my six-day visit, I vividly experienced her pervading compassionate presence. She was there in the rocky ocean caves and on the long gentle beaches. She was expressed in the sea wind, the warmth of rock and sand, the buzzing of cicadas in the bushes, and *in me*.

In Oakland, now, a month later, I sat in Mountain View Cemetery under a huge, venerable tree and I visualized her. She began as a figure outside myself. I saw her in detail, situated in the full moon above the ocean, and opened myself to her energy of compassion. I visualized Kwan Yin closer and closer until she merged with me, and I felt her presence strongly inside me. Through the meditation, distinctions between inner and outer dissolved, letting me experience a blissful unity with all life. Then gradually, Kwan Yin became separate again, grew smaller and smaller until she disappeared, and I was left resting in my own nature, feeling strongly connected with myself.

"Please hold me in these coming days," I said aloud. "Please help me to be completely in my experience, bravely, realistically.

"Please help me to be always considerate and kind to the people who are coming to help me, and grateful to them.

"Please help me to be large enough to contain what is going to happen to me, and keep my center.

"Please help me to be with Crystal, who is frightened that I'm going to die and leave her. Help me not to be impatient with her or to participate in her pessimism and fear."

The day before, we had fought as Crystal made demands on me that I could not understand. She had insisted I purchase life insurance. She did not, she told me, want to be "left holding the bag" if I died. She did not want to be responsible for my funeral costs. And she wanted to be paid back the money I owed her. In the preceding years, I had made payments on a loan to Crystal, but had done so only sporadically and casually. Yet she had watched me raise a large sum of money for my trip to China, and knew that if I had wanted to repay her I could have easily done so. By the time I had returned from China, she was filled up with hurt and resentment, an accumulation of four years of unresolved feelings. Now, to hear that she might have to take even more financial responsibility drove her to the edge. Looking ahead, she anticipated that she might have to use her own resources to care for me; she wanted me to express my concern for her by preparing for the possibility of my death. Again, our differences caused us pain: our needs were not the same. What I needed Crystal to say to me was, "You are my precious person. I'm afraid you will die and leave me." What she needed me to say to her was, "I know this will be hard for you financially, let me at least make sure you're taken care of if I die." Instead, each of us felt the other did not understand our respective needs and did not care, and we withdrew from one another.

Now I asked Kwan Yin to help me to be compassionate to Crystal, to understand her fears and consider her needs even as I began the struggle for my own survival. I hoped we could regain some closeness.

The air felt cold against my cheeks and a little damp, as though rain might be coming. I could hear the winglike branches of the tall palms clashing against each other in the breeze.

A tiny plane arched across the sky from the direction of the Oakland airport. Ruth Denison had talked once about standing down in the desert looking up at an airplane and thinking about the people sitting in the passenger section, drinking their drinks, eating their food, alive in a whole different world. I felt like that now. I had passed over into another realm, like the novelist Harold Brodkey describing his AIDS diagnosis: "I felt...as if I had been invited, almost abducted, to a party, a somber feast not entirely grim, a feast of the seriously afflicted." I was now as separate from others as the people in the airplane now passing overhead were separate from me. All those who had not yet been invited to the "feast of the seriously afflicted" existed at a distance from me. Even though I knew the division was artificial, I felt my imprisonment in this particular body that would soon be subjected to grotesquely intrusive maneuvers.

I was at the center of something now: people in my community were mobilizing to help me. I was *the one* this time. As much as the others were with me, I was still alone in that center where everything pointed at me. I had to meet this aloneness, and immerse myself deeply in it so that it could become a place in which we shared—whether the others knew it or not—our humanness and our fear of death. Sick or well, all of us participate in the Buddha's First Noble Truth, the truth of suffering, and we create our suffering by clinging to feelings and experiences, to people and objects, trying to forge something permanent of that which is always shifting and changing.

Perhaps I should just prepare for death, I thought, just believe that I was going to die during the surgery on Thursday morning. To prepare, I would want to be fully present in every moment until then. Starting now: for this wind that was blowing across my skin, the kitsch of the monuments here in the cemetery, and the trees—especially the trees. They were singing to me, strummed by the wind. I wanted to have such a clear, intensely calm experience right now that if I died on the way home it would be all right. But then I thought about the hospital, and realized that it was one thing to sit up here with so much space and beauty around me, and say that I could let my spirit go; it would be quite another to be in a hospital surrounded by machines, injected with chemicals, invaded in ways that were meant to be helpful but were nonetheless terrifying. To lie down on this grass and let oneself go—that would be a peaceful end.

As it became darker and colder, the clouds massing above, I found myself chanting, *"Namo Guan Shih Yin pusa,"* the Chinese invocation to Kwan Yin. She saves us from disaster; she arrives in many guises to pluck people from burning buildings, to calm the ocean storms and rescue the sailors. As I chanted, I felt her in everything, the way I had on the beach at Putuo Shan: in the grass beneath me, in the breeze on my skin, in the distant mutter of traffic, and in my own body. In my colon. Kwan Yin was there in the tumor too—even there. Could I understand that each of the doctors was Kwan Yin, and each of the surgeons? The anesthesiologist? All of the nurses? Couldn't they all be Kwan Yin?

As I chanted, asking for Kwan Yin's help, I sensed that my voice, my plea, my question, reached somewhere and was received. It reached deep inside *me*, past preoccupations of self, and touched a silent place that exists independent of struggle and fear, that place of deep quiet that I had experienced in meditation—a place as empty and free of boundaries as the sky.

Pema Chodron, Buddhist teacher and nun, says, "By looking directly into our own heart, we find the awakened Buddha, the completely unclouded experience of how things really are."

Under a spreading tree, beneath a cloud-clotted sky. I felt the aliveness of everything around me, and my own body and mind sharing in that life. And I knew my separation, too. "Help me," I said, and felt how utterly alone I was, like a tiny figure skimpy against a vast horizon. And yet Kwan Yin answered, awakening a resonance as deep in me as the core of the huge tree under which I sat. I dropped into that place of resonance, and found myself willing to experience what I must.

3

Dhamma Dena, 1981

Cultivate the healing power of the pure unattached mind.
Ruth Denison

MY SPIRITUAL PRACTICE was inaugurated two decades ago in the Mojave
Desert. A friend drove us there—ten hours south from Oakland, through
the little town of Joshua Tree, and up a long desert slope to Copper
Mountain Mesa, where, along a sandy dirt road, we came to a cluster of
low buildings huddled under the killer sun. Here I first met Ruth Denison, a German-born woman trained in the Burmese tradition of Theravada Buddhism. Ruth's flexibility and sense of what Westerners need in
order to practice mindfulness had led her to develop a challenging teaching style grounded in traditional practice and augmented with her own
innovations. She was known as a creative teacher, who would employ
any means to communicate her beloved "Dharma"; she was also the first
Buddhist teacher to offer women-only retreats.

Another person might have approached meditation gradually, carefully, beginning with short sessions of a few minutes each day and slowly
graduating to longer periods of sitting; this would be the sane way to
proceed. But I had plunged in, signing up right away for a seven-day
silent meditation retreat—a regime in which we rose at 6 A.M., meditated, ate, returned for the morning session of sitting and walking meditation, ate, rested, returned in the afternoon for more sitting and walking
meditation, ate, returned in the evening to listen to a "Dharma talk" from
Ruth, followed by more meditation, and then went to bed, to rise again
at 6 A.M.

The silence, observed by everyone but Ruth, who guided the meditations and gave evening "Dharma talks," was difficult for me, since it made me feel unseen, unacknowledged. It seemed that people had become zombies, walking slowly with solemn faces and avoiding eye contact with other human beings. I found this especially painful with the friend who had brought me there. Normally we chattered together, commiserated, and joked. Now she looked past me as if I did not exist. It wasn't until the end of the week that I began to experience the benefits of the silence and lack of conventional social contact. In this vacuum, I observed my conditioned impulse to reach out, to engage another person or get their attention. In the absence of this stimulation I was left with only myself, stewing in my worries and self-deprecating or self-aggrandizing comparisons, my remembered hurts, my sense of inadequacy. At first this was excruciating, but as the week progressed, I found myself grateful to be experiencing my own thoughts and sensations without the distraction of other people's opinions of me and responses to me. Sometimes a sadness would well up, and I would feel warm tears running down my face; sometimes I felt a great wounded tenderness for myself, as though I were watching a child struggling to accomplish a too difficult task; now and then an expansive peacefulness opened in my chest and I found myself smiling. The silence had become my friend.

I returned once or twice a year to retreats in the desert to learn from Ruth Denison, and also began to meditate at home. Over the years Ruth's meditation center—named Dhamma Dena for a distinguished female teacher from the Buddha's lifetime (Dhammadinna)—became the cradle in which my timid beginning attempts at awareness were rocked and nurtured. I learned that the practice Ruth taught, called *vipassana* or insight meditation, came from the Theravada Buddhist tradition. Not the famous Zen, with its poetry and spare esthetics, nor the exotic Tibetan Buddhism with its world-renowned Dalai Lama, Theravada Buddhism is original Buddhism, its practices taught by the Buddha 2,500 years ago in India and pursued now in Southeast Asian countries. Theravada is known as the gradual path, involving effort made through many lifetimes toward the goal of liberation from suffering. It emphasizes "bare attention" and "choiceless awareness," teaching a method for being wholly present in one's own experience, without censoring or denying anything.

Through this method one arrives at an understanding of the three marks of existence: *dukkha,* or suffering; *anicca,* or impermanence; and *anatta,* or the unreality of the individual self. "Individual existence, as well as the whole world," wrote Theravada monk Nyanatiloka, "are in reality nothing but a process of ever-changing phenomena which are comprised in the Five Groups of Existence." Everything, in other words, is a temporary compound, always subject to change—human beings ourselves being a collection of material and immaterial faculties that function together for a time and then fall apart at death. These faculties "in no way constitute a real Ego-entity or subsisting personality, and equally no self, soul or substance can be found outside of these groups as their 'owner.'" One example is a house, which is built of various materials, but has no "house"-identity separate from those compounded elements. The Buddha said that all existence is like this, empty of a permanent self or substance. In vipassana meditation, one becomes aware of the ever-changing nature of one's own sensations and perceptions and begins to see through the illusion of a stable self. Suffering occurs when one tries to hold on to pleasant feelings or pull away from pain. Liberation would come if one were able to fully realize and embrace the experience of the phenomenal world's constant shifting and changing. This is the goal of the Buddha's teaching.

Theravada Buddhism was established in the United States mostly by Westerners, young people who studied in Burma, Thailand, or Sri Lanka and brought the practice back with them in order to pass it on to their peers in America. Ruth Denison, somewhat older than the others, had journeyed to Burma with her American husband, studied and practiced there, and received "transmission" from a noted Burmese Buddhist master. Although her teacher, U Ba Khin, had authorized Ruth to teach meditation, she had been modest about her capacities; upon her return to the United States she had steadily pursued her meditation practice both alone and in Zen centers in Los Angeles (at that time there were no Theravada centers in Southern California), but did not set out to teach. She and her husband hosted spiritual teachers in their Hollywood home and were part of a circle of seekers including Alan Watts and Timothy Leary. Eventually, students began to gather around Ruth, asking her to teach them to meditate. They followed her to the desert, and the center now called Dhamma Dena was born in several tiny buildings.

From the beginning of my visits to Dhamma Dena, the stark, spacious environment made a vibrant container for the practice. My memory holds many vivid encounters with the desert and Ruth, like one particular morning in the early eighties when I had used the break after breakfast to hide away behind the work shed and write in my journal. (Reading and writing are discouraged at meditation retreats.)

The sun blazed down upon me while I leaned over my notebook, now and then glancing up at the flat tan earth and the sage and creosote bushes bobbing in the wind. Yellow blossoms adorned the creosote bushes in this brief desert spring. Out across the land, a few tiny houses lay scattered; distant rounded mountains like sleeping elephants marked the horizon.

A rich deep sound filled the sky, awakening a throbbing in my body. This guttural song came at intervals throughout the day, a motif to remind us where we were: the stretch of dry earth extending out before me was near the Marine Corps Base at Twentynine Palms, not far from the Flight Test Center at Edwards Air Force Base; and to the north were the U.S. Naval Weapons Center, the Irwin Military Reservation, and the Randsburg Wash Test Range. The desert in its vastness is conducive to meditation, it is so open and still; these sounds of jets and explosions punched holes in the silence, reminding us of mortality.

Here in the high desert on Copper Mountain Mesa, just north of Joshua Tree National Monument, suffering and impermanence were close companions. A shirt left outside for two weeks is eaten by the sun, its cotton hanging in shreds; an unwanted dog thrown out of a passing car may wander in confusion and hunger until it steps into the cruel jaws of a trap set for small animals; plants shrivel, skin dries and creases, eyes are stunned by the flashbulb-intensity of the sun.

I was picking up my notebook and readying myself to leave my private place behind the shed when a long-skirted figure appeared from around the woodpile. Ruth was short and square-shouldered, her hair covered by a tucked white scarf, her long-sleeved white blouse and tan skirt fluttering against her body in the wind. On her face was an expression of satisfaction as she looked down at the desert tortoise clasped in her hands. Behind her waddled an ancient dachshund who accompanied his steps with a deep throaty cough as he hurried to catch up.

"Ah, this is where you are hiding!" For a moment Ruth stopped and stood looking at me, as though she could not decide whether to talk to me or go on about her business. The tortoise swam in the air energetically, its head thrust out of the shell.

Ruth grinned down at it.

"Look at her! I found her caught in the junk pile, yah, in the wire under there. She couldn't move. I come out here sometimes just to check on her."

She held the tortoise for me to see.

It was about the size of a small round casserole dish, its grayish shell like joined plates of mail, each section outlined in darker gray. Its head wagged from side to side, and as Ruth set it gently on the earth, its legs scrabbled for traction, pushing its weight forward on horny toenails.

In Buddhist lore, the turtle and the elephant are symbols of mindfulness: they move slowly and deliberately, looking down at the ground and surveying all as they walk.

"She is hungry!" Ruth said, folding her hands before her. "I am going to take her to the house and give her some salad."

The dog came up to peer at the turtle with its old bluish eyes, and I smiled, remembering Ruth's remark yesterday about the tufts of black hair above its eyes. "Special eyebrows," she had said, smoothing the strands of coarse hair. "I call them the Suzuki eyebrows. Have you ever seen a picture of that great Zen scholar D. T. Suzuki? He had eyebrows that *stuck* into the universe." She had paused, surveying the dog's face. "Yah, they formed an umbrella over his eyes."

Now the dog, whose name was Uliloo, sought out the shade under the overhang of a makeshift wooden platform someone had built to support a mattress. Only his shaggy brown muzzle poked out, alternately pointing from the tortoise to Ruth.

"Want to sit down?" I asked, moving over to accommodate her.

"No, darling, I have many things to do. I must get back up to the house and then we have a sitting at nine, hmm?"

But instead of hurrying off, she stooped down, her skirt spreading over the dry yellow dirt, to stroke Uliloo's head. "He's really a sweetheart, you know. He's not supposed to eat now because he's going to the vet. He's looking at me. You see how dependent animals are? He cannot speak. The desire is in front of him: to eat. And he can only look at me, he can't be angry, he can't take anything for himself. You see, the dependency is enormous. We are not aware of it. But this feeling only comes when you really begin to see the suffering in the world."

Uliloo flopped on his side, panting so heavily that he began to choke again. The choking accelerated into a coughing fit in which he became the perfect embodiment of suffering. This old dog had a heart condition, his lungs and bronchial tubes filling with liquid. I watched sympathetically, accustomed to this distress by now, as Ruth fussed over him, stroking him tenderly, urging him to relax.

After his last paroxysm, Uliloo fell back in exhaustion, grunting rhythmically to himself.

Ruth perched on the edge of the platform and, shaking her head, looked with great solicitude at the dog. She was a sixty-year-old woman with a strong-boned, lined face. Her bangs, visible beneath the edges of the scarf, were dull blond, touched with red. During the first year I had meditated with Ruth Denison I never saw her without one of those little scarves tucked up in the back, and eventually I began to wonder if she were bald. But actually, she had long hair twisted up under the scarf. "Not a gray hair in it," she had told me. "In my family we do not get gray." Once, on a visit to the Women's Sangha in Berkeley she had worn a deep-colored dress and let her hair down over her shoulders. The effect was startling; she looked as vulnerable as a young girl.

Now her eyes squinted against the sun, the dark eyebrows above the deep sockets furrowed, her bright blue gaze shadowed. Her jaw was a proud hull, her face a ship cutting through turbulent waters.

She had lost all incentive to get back to the house now, I saw, for she was looking at the objects in a pile near us, no doubt devising a use for each. Behind us was a junkyard of old wood, shiny household appliances, coiled wire, doors of various shapes, casement windows, and pieces of metal, all neatly stacked or propped in rows and piles: the detritus of the desert, gathered from abandoned houses or bought for almost nothing from past settlers who had decided to give up and go back to Los Angeles or San Bernardino, where the sun was not so blistering or the wind so vicious. "Gifts from the universe," Ruth called these objects.

I was feeling grumpy and tired, having struggled through the early morning meditation session and afterwards castigated myself that I was not really a very religious or spiritual person. Ruth, on the other hand, had always been drawn to religious practice. As a child in Germany, she was devoted to the church and loved to pray. She had even been attracted to her American husband because he was so "spiritual," having been a monk in the Hindu tradition of Vedanta. Adjusting my stiffening buttocks on my makeshift seat of piled boards, I looked over at Ruth, who had picked up a piece of rusted metal and sat examining it with the shrewd eye of one who can devise a use for anything.

We began to talk about how Ruth had come to offer all-women retreats. She alternated them now with her general retreats, attended by both men and women.

"Certainly I am a woman who is not totally dependent on the man," Ruth said. "Before I married I was very independent; I was a schoolteacher and a principal. When I married, I just took that wifely role for a while because I didn't need to work. But as you can see, I didn't stay in that role, so there is some blood in me. But I must say, I have one quality that is remarkable, which is, I have no need for revenge." She had told us before about her experiences during World War II in Germany, when she was raped and violently handled, but she obviously harbored no bitterness.

Ruth continued: "In many ways I have brought good karma forces with me, with natural balance, with a sense of justice coming from a deeper soul or ground, and a great compassionate feeling. I have a love for life, hmm? Which brings with it sensitivity and care, *real* care. So when you have that certain sense you cannot really charge back, no matter how wrong what was done to you. Because when you charge back, you see that you injure life, and the principle is not injuring life."

I had seen Ruth work tirelessly to create and maintain this center in which people could meditate and learn to know themselves, to practice how to be present to life, how to allow each life-form to realize its full cycle and potential. She cherished the cactus plant in the dry dirt yard and watched each year as a small bird returned to its nest among the spines and raised its babies there. She cleaned and repaired, tended the physical environment, and fed the rabbits and coyotes when food was scarce. And she gave endlessly to her students, always seeking ways to wake us up to our own joy and beauty. I felt something celebratory in all this, some large and joyful possibility of living in harmony with all of existence.

Later I watched Ruth stride briskly away, the tortoise held out before her. Uliloo struggled up on his legs to follow. In this headlong flight, her body tilted slightly forward and her skirt billowing about her legs, Ruth looked like one of the factory women in a Kaethe Kollwitz lithograph, someone strong-armed and resilient, whose life is labor.

I stood thinking about the concept she had articulated. To promote life, to nurture and celebrate it, even my own life—to get out of my way and enjoy the show.

Pondering that possibility, I walked slowly back to Dukkha House, the women's dormitory.

For two days now, in the concrete-block meditation hall, we had been cultivating mindfulness. The whole endeavor of meditation is to become aware of what is going on, right here and now. You would only have to sit down in silence for a short while to realize that this is not easy, for we usually reside either in the future or the past, our monkey minds jumping around to everywhere but here. Remembering, planning, worrying, longing, regretting, we distract ourselves endlessly from our actual sensations of living. Where does life take place? It happens in our bodies, our feelings, in the workings and contents of our minds. In our effort to develop awareness, we begin with the body, which is called the First Foundation of Mindfulness.

I was to learn that in traditional Theravada practice, the meditator spends two years focusing intensively and only on mindfulness of the body before moving on to the other foundations of mindfulness, in this methodical way becoming aware of the true nature of her own human existence. This practice, it is said, "causes the world to appear."

Ruth rang the bell for us to begin the meditation. I sat with my legs crossed and my back as straight as I could make it, and closed my eyes. Ruth's voice directed us to pay attention to the motion of our breathing. This, she told us, was the air element that we share with all living creatures, that sustains our life, never stopping from the time we draw our first breath until life goes out of us. And yet we are almost never aware of this constant activity. Focusing upon it now, she assured us, could help us to concentrate and calm our minds.

One location to do this, she told us, was the belly, which expands with each in-breath and then returns to normal. As this is a fairly gross motion, it is a good object of concentration.

So I directed myself to be aware of the pushing out of my belly as I breathed in, and its flattening as I breathed out. For a few breaths all went well, as I trained my consciousness on this simple bodily movement.

Then my mind flew to my apartment in Oakland and I began to wonder whether the person who had promised to feed my cat was doing so. Had I made the instructions explicit enough? Had I....

"If your mind has wandered,"—Ruth's voice from the front of the room—"gently bring it back to your focus on the breath."

With a shock I realized how far I had gone away from this body and this room. Even though I had been doing this meditation for a year, still I found it difficult to maintain concentration. Humbly I brought my attention back to the movement of my belly.

Now Ruth directed us to be aware of our nostrils, feeling the sensations of the air passing over our upper lip, in and out. She asked us not to manipulate our breathing, making it deeper or shallower, but simply to observe it.

I began to be able to hold my focus, and felt my breath slowing and becoming subtler.

In my first few retreats at Dhamma Dena, I had sometimes peeked at the other meditators, seeing a man sitting very still and erect, a woman in a long skirt who smiled as she meditated, and I had thought *they* must *really* know how to do this! My heart would sink as I suspected that this practice was not for me, that it was a mistake to have come; I would never be able to sit so serenely. Now, I knew that the person sitting in such perfect posture might be raging inside or spinning out in flights of imagination, indulging in sexual fantasies, or, as Ruth put it, simply "hanging out in Lala-land." And I had discovered that each time I sat down to meditate, I encountered a new situation. It was impossible to predict what I would experience, and therefore I had to surrender to the reality of each moment as I strove to develop concentration.

From the front of the room, Ruth spoke again. "If you find yourself thinking, realize that you are thinking—and it will even help if you say to yourself, 'thinking.' Then gently return your attention to the breath.

"Let your breath express itself naturally," Ruth reminded us. "You are the observer only, you don't need to participate. The body breathes by itself."

With all the care I could muster, I brought my consciousness to my physical being, to feel the touch of the breath on my upper lip.

So the forty-five minute session went, back and forth from concentrating on my breath to worries and frustration. Ruth's quiet voice called me once again to pay attention; each time I reminded myself that I had been "thinking" or "worrying" or "remembering," and brought my attention back to my breath.

In the final five minutes I peeked at the clock, and then I felt that I could not endure even one more second of this stillness. My body tightened and twitched, wanting to get up and shake itself. Surreptitiously watching the slender hand on my watch-face jolt from second to second, I tortured myself with every increment of time's slow passing.

When the bell finally rang at the front of the room, I realized how utterly I had abandoned my concentration.

"Now in the space before the final bell," Ruth directed, "please recollect what you are doing and recommit yourself to your mindfulness of the breath."

Given this second chance, I returned my attention to my upper lip to feel the passage of my breath again. My mind came to rest there, and I focused.

The final bell rang. Placing my hands before me on the rug, I bowed, acknowledging my own effort and expressing my gratitude for the opportunity to practice.

I looked up to see Ruth sitting before us, relaxed and welcoming. She smiled with a knowing tenderness that brought tears to my eyes.

"Now you have experienced *dukkha*," she said. "The Buddha's First Noble Truth, as it is expressed in the Pali language, *dukkha*—the truth of suffering. Because we are human beings, we suffer; because we cling to pleasant sensations and try to push away the unpleasant ones, we suffer.

"And you have realized impermanence—how everything constantly flows and changes. You have noticed this with each breath, no? How it begins with the in-breath, comes to its completion, and dies with the out-breath. Then another breath must come. This is the truth of all life— that it is constantly coming into being and falling away—even our own precious bodies. This is the truth of impermanence that the Buddha taught."

She sat looking out at us, letting the silence settle around her words. Then an encouraging smile lit her face.

"So you see, you have penetrated into the deep teachings of Buddhism. I congratulate your beautiful selves on your excellent sitting meditation."

4

Mother Highland

Joy is exactly what's happening minus our opinion of it.
Joko Beck

I HAD NEVER STAYED OVERNIGHT in a hospital. I had had operations for a broken arm and an injured knee, but afterward had been able to go home to recuperate in my own bedroom. As an employee—secretary to a heart doctor in a San Francisco medical center and transcriptionist in the pathology laboratory in another hospital—I had thought of myself as doing useful work, much more in line with the Buddhist idea of "right livelihood" than my previous stints at an auto leasing firm and an insurance company. Dressed in a starched white coat, I had logged in specimens, typed insurance forms, and walked briskly down the hospital corridors carrying file folders or jars of body parts recently removed in the operating room. My work had been several steps removed from the patient who lay in bed.

Now my position had shifted, and I had the awful sense of being the one caught in the center of the spider web. Time seemed to be narrowing, moving inexorably to that moment when they would wheel me into the operating room and cut me open. Most of all I dreaded the anesthetic, that plunge downward into the black hole of unconsciousness, the utter helplessness from which I might or might not rise up again.

As Crystal and I drove out the morning freeway, the traffic on our side was sparse, while the commute west to the Bay Bridge and San Francisco, going the other direction, moved in a molasses-slow stream of cars. The freeway wound out into East Oakland, the wooded hills of the wealthy rising to our left and the flat lands of the ordinary folks spreading to our right down toward the bay. Soon, ahead of us, we could see the bulk of

Highland Hospital above the hilly streets of houses. It's like a military bunker, I thought, looking at the gray concrete fortress; it's like the Pentagon.

"How long do you think it'll be before they take you in?" Crystal asked. Not an early riser, she had a blurry undefined look about her this morning.

"No telling. They explained to me—if someone gets brought in for an emergency, everyone else has to wait. They just want you to come there early so you'll be available."

At my feet rested Crystal's bag with her lined music paper, her unfinished score.

As we pulled into a parking space several blocks from the hospital, I took a long deep breath. Yes this is really happening, I told myself. You really are going to go through this surgery.

The pre-operation room had a low ceiling and was dimly lit, with a bright island of the nurses' station at its center. In my hospital gown, on a high bed, I was wheeled into place in the line of bodies waiting to be taken through the swinging doors into the several operating rooms. A kindly nurse inserted a needle in my hand to attach me to a bag of fluids on an IV pole. She pulled up a chair for Crystal, and returned to her station at the center of the room.

Then we waited. Crystal was attentive, engaging me in gentle conversation, until I told her it was really all right for her to work on her music. Then she pulled her score out of her bag, positioned it on her lap, and bent over it. As I had neither my glasses nor anything to read, I had nothing to do but watch the wall clock in its slow progression and observe the activity in the room. The other patients lay still, one man with his hands folded across his chest and eyes staring upward. The nurses wrote on clipboards, talked into phones, and consulted with doctors wearing green smocks.

After some time, Crystal and I agreed that an hour had passed. Maybe I would be next. No one had yet been wheeled out of the room. "Can I do anything for you?" she asked. "Well," I answered uncertainly, "I'm not sure my IV is working." We both peered steadily at the clear plastic bag on its pole. No drip. "Let me get the nurse," Crystal said. She put down her papers and went to the nurses' station; there she talked with someone who turned to look at me. Not until my IV had been adjusted did Crystal return to working on her score.

Relieved, I lay watching a muscular male nurse tend to the patient next to me.

Okay, I told myself, how about just breathing? As I had done at Dhamma Dena and so many mornings in my own home, I brought my attention to my breath, feeling the warmth of my belly under my hands, feeling it rise and fall. Stop waiting, I told myself, this can be meditation time; and soon I was able to concentrate for a short while, entering a state of calm, hearing the noises in the room but not being distracted by them.

Another hour passed. The man in the corpse pose was wheeled through the double doors. I thought of calling out, "Hey, good luck! Bon voyage! Break a leg!"

Then, lying there, I became acutely aware that my body was going to be offered up to the knife, as though I were an Aztec maiden on a mountaintop. Funny how life gives us the opportunity to play all the roles.

"God, Crystal," I said, to distract myself from such thoughts, "it's been three hours already!"

She looked up, and I watched her come out of her concentration, shifting her attention away from the music. "Has it?" she asked, glancing up at the clock.

Wanting to comfort me, she began to tell me about all the people who had called to express concern. "We're going to have a meeting tomorrow at the house to talk about how people can help with your care. The Wandering Menstruals are organizing it."

"Yes?" I tried to focus my attention on her words, to pull away from the anxious space of this waiting room, the prone bodies, and the prospect that awaited me.

"And they'll all come see you in the hospital. You're going to have lots of visitors."

"Yeah," I nodded absently, and gave up the effort to imagine the scene. My friends existed in a universe separate from the small sounds and muted voices, the chrome and glass of this room.

Lying back again, I tried to summon my life, the life that had engaged me so strongly with the people Crystal named. While growing up, I had learned so many ways of holding myself apart from others that I came to exist inside a fortress, alternately comforting myself with illusions of superiority and torturing myself with convictions of inferiority. This emotional and psychic vacuum had propelled me to a dead end. In my early thirties, married, busily employed at a job and writing, apparently happy, I would awake on a Saturday morning and be unable to rise from bed. My husband would be in the next room puttering with his ham radio, as I floated in a gray fog.

Lying in bed, pondering my life, I had realized that going it alone had not worked. I needed other people. Yet I knew that they could save me only if I were willing to tear down my fortress and emerge without defenses, a prospect that made my heart flutter with terror. One day my husband had snapped angrily at me, "Sandy, why don't you join the human race!?" The next Saturday morning as I was again lying in bed unable to move, I knew that I must either join the human race or perish, because so much in me had already withered; and if I didn't save the rest I would surely die.

I found the Women's Liberation movement of the early seventies, in which women came together to change their lives and create a humane future for all people. I joined a "consciousness raising" group, where women spoke about their lives. Taking my turn, with great awkwardness, and trembling with a fear that turned my gut to jelly, I forced myself to tell the story of my life to a roomful of strangers, exposing myself as I had never done before. I left all judgments behind as I heard the other women's hopes and fears, their struggles to survive, to do meaningful work and be recognized for it, to support their children and raise them well.

Sometimes in the meetings, as people shared their pain and their aspirations, or in the demonstrations (or "actions" as we called them) in which we confronted the institutions that denied and restricted women and children, I would feel lifted in a sense of communion so strong that it could only be called spiritual—it was a belonging, not just to this group of women but to all humanity, and awakened in me a sense of responsibility and tenderness for every human being alive. I had found a way to join the human race, and this activism became my spiritual practice for ten years. It was a natural movement outward from my personal concerns to a general responsiveness to all life. When I came to Buddhism at the beginning of the eighties, there was much that I already understood, and I combined my spiritual practice with political work. Meditation and the practice of sending loving-kindness to all beings helped me to ground myself in provocative situations and avoid the violent activism that mirrored the tactics of the oppressor.

In my life generally, my Buddhist practice helped me meet difficulties and work my way through crises, functioning as a rudder that kept me on course even through the bumpiest seas. It gave me ways to be aware of what I was feeling and experiencing, to stay connected to the deep certainty of life's interpenetration and continuation.

Now the cancer would teach me how it felt to need others in a crucial, life-sustaining way. The friends Crystal had mentioned were people with whom I had worked, meditated, lived, and played. We had shared our lives in ways that strongly connected us, so it made sense to them to step forward to help me.

In the pre-op room I let go of that other life outside, trusting that it would return sometime after this fateful day. My life now was here in this room, my body more and more restless from lying in the bed, and my mind wandering except during the brief periods when I could calm it and focus on my breath.

Another hour passed. Another patient was wheeled away.

The nurse came to pat my ankle. "Sorry you're having to wait so long."

When she had gone, I turned on my side, careful of the needle in my hand, and lay watching Crystal pore over the big pages of her score, checking the endless details involved in a work that employed many instruments and voices. I thought about how much had changed since those early years together when we touched each other at every opportunity and made love eagerly. We had shared so many dimensions of our lives: supporting each other in our work, traveling, hiking, going out to music and dance performances. While watching the Alvin Ailey or Merce Cunningham dance companies, we would become so stimulated by the beautiful moving bodies that we would rush home to make love, laughing at ourselves. In the winters we would drive to Lake Tahoe to cross-country ski, and in the snowy landscape Crystal would transform. Her carefulness of herself, her reticence, would fall away, and she became energetic and joyful, generously helping me in my awkward beginner's efforts to ski. Now and then her daughter came to visit us, and we developed a warm relationship. Crystal bought the house in Oakland, making sure that both of us had space to work at home. We had built a life together of routines and structures that served us both, gave us pleasure, and supported us in difficult times. I had trusted the deep connection I had felt in the meadow at Vallecitos, and had known that I was fully committed to this union.

Yet over time our fights about money, about our different approaches to life, my impatience, and her fear of my anger, caused us to withdraw, both physically and emotionally. Gradually the intimacy drained out of our many shared activities until we barely touched each other; we had not made love for over a year. I was still attracted to Crystal, but I could not cross the distance to her.

She had also been feeling very unsatisfied with our relationship, she later told me. While I was in China, she had looked at our life and felt that she was the one who gave more, at least materially, having lent me money and set up a comfortable house in which I paid rent and did some maintenance work, but did not take as much responsibility as she did. The years of unresolved conflict came to a head, arousing her anger and her conviction that something crucial must change. She felt used by me, and resolved that unless I took more responsibility for the house and paid off my debt to her, our relationship might end.

When I returned from China, Crystal did not communicate her needs to me, busy as she was with her composing, and so I did not know that the structure of our shared life was creaking and shuddering. Then the cancer arrived—brutal and unavoidable—and the gulfs in our relationship suddenly seemed unbridgeable.

When the orderly came to unlock the wheels of my bed, Crystal looked up, her blue eyes wide with alarm. "This is it," I said. She stood, clutching her score to her chest, and for a moment we stared into each other's eyes. Then I was being wheeled beneath the white soundproof-tile ceiling. I heard the double doors swing open, and I knew for sure that it was too late to leap from the bed, rip out the needle, and run!

When I awoke that evening—or partially awoke, for I drifted in a morphine fog—it was as Crystal had predicted. Familiar faces floated before me, hands touched my arm and squeezed my foot somewhere down at the end of the bed. Bouquets had arrived and cards were taped to the yellowish wall. The room in which I was lying was small, and behind a curtain next to my bed, I knew dimly, another person was lying. Laughter and music from a TV set dominated the atmosphere, loud noises entered from the hallway. The nurses scurried about. My friends had had to talk their way in to see me, they told me; it was like an armed camp down in the lobby, with guards screening every visitor. Each of them had insisted, "I'm her sister!" in order to be allowed past the pistol-toting guard to come up to the seventh floor and crowd in here with me.

"You sure have a lot of sisters," the nurse remarked.

That night my student Deborah stayed all night with me, and answered some of my questions about the hospital. "No, Sandy, not all hospitals are like this." I figured she must know, since she worked as a nurse at the University of California medical center hospital in San Francisco. She chuckled, glancing around her. "Really, this is a circus in comparison to most."

Deborah is a large woman with brown hair that falls straight down her back. She speaks in the sweet slow accents of North Carolina, as if she is savoring the words in the back of her mouth, sucking off the edges so they come out mellow and smooth as caramel.

Deborah helped me into a chair and sponged me with a cloth soaked in water and eucalyptus-scented soap that she had brought from home. Avoiding the eight-inch open incision that bisected my belly, being careful of the IV needle, and watching out for the tube that entered through my nose and snaked down inside to drain brown acids from my stomach, she drew the soft wet rag over my skin. My body, so utterly vulnerable now after the assault of surgery, slowly surrendered to her touch. I felt a deep, voluptuous pleasure, enhanced by the awareness that I was alive still, that my body could feel something pleasurable. When Deborah had toweled me dry, she changed the linen on my hospital bed, helped me back into it, and pulled the clean-smelling sheet up over my chest.

Perhaps Kwan Yin had arrived yet again, speeding from her South China island to inhabit Deborah's body and guide her gentle hands. There is so much lore centered on Kwan Yin's hands and arms: the thousand-armed Kwan Yin ready to reach out and avert every disaster, grant every wish; the celebrated Princess Miao Shan who gave up her arms and eyes to save her father's life; the statue missing its right arm that traveled across the sea to a little village and prevailed on a carpenter there to carve the goddess a new arm.

But Deborah knew nothing of these stories: she wanted to have a conversation about literature. Through my morphine haze, I marshaled the meager brain power available to me, and we talked of writing and writers. Then I fell asleep seeing Deborah's round kind face smiling at me.

The afternoon of the day after my surgery, visiting hours brought quite a number of people to see my roommate, an African-American woman. On my side of the curtain that separated us several of my friends had also crowded in. The TV set blared. In the hallway, doors banged, and people talked loudly. I huddled in the bed, thinking to myself, "I cannot bear this." The morphine made me feel besieged, not able to protect myself or find a psychic place in which to rest.

I had imagined that morphine would make me high—maybe a little like grass or acid (substances I had not imbibed in years). But it was not like any experience I had had. Somewhere in my lower body there was pain, and morphine was a blessed steel door that kept it contained. But it also made me feel disconnected from everything around me. I struggled to *get here*—into this room, this moment—but couldn't quite make it. Particularly as a meditator committed to being as fully present as possible, I experienced this dislocation as a moment-by-moment deprivation. Worse, because of the effects of the drug, I was completely at the mercy of every sound, every sight, and every jolt—everything in the environment; I had no way to filter anything out. So a door slamming in the hall, the sound of the TV, people's voices, someone knocking against my bed—all of that entered and assaulted me. The morphine had so stripped away my powers that I could not call upon my practice to ground me in this setting, or perhaps the failure was mine in not being able to surrender to it. I was resisting the morphine and the environment, wanting them to be different rather than letting them be as they were and exploring my experience of them.

The hospital social worker had arrived. She and Crystal were discussing the ins and outs of applying for public medical assistance across my bed. Another visitor, a young woman named Corbin who had been a student of mine, moved toward the bed, and suddenly tangled her feet in the base of my IV stand. The stand tipped, and before she could catch it, the needle attaching me to the fluid-bag jerked in my hand. I gasped and winced, looking up into Corbin's eyes as she realized what she had done, and I saw that she was horrified at her clumsiness.

Corbin and I gazed helplessly at each other. It seemed we were caught in equal distress. The moment was made surreal by Crystal's and the social worker's obliviousness to it. I could see that Corbin wanted a way to apologize and did not know what to do, so I asked, "Corbin, could you rub my back?" She nodded and stepped forward, this time ever so carefully skirting the IV stand, and I turned on my side. As she began to massage my back, pushing into the muscles, I objected, "No, please just stroke it." Then we were enclosed in an intimacy, Corbin with slow strokes moving her warm hand from shoulder to hip down my back.

Crystal and the counselor continued discussing health care strategy as I struggled to pay attention to Corbin's touch. Her awkwardness had left her, and the hand that touched me felt strong and sure. Now and then it came to rest and for a few moments simply held me. In my morphine fog, I brought my attention as much as I could to the contact between Corbin's skin and mine, and gradually that place of warmth gave me knowledge of our connection: two living beings, not separate, breathing together, skins touching and warmth shared. Then Corbin would begin to stroke again, her hand gliding slowly down toward my lower back, spreading that sense of connection until it calmed my whole body. My breath was somewhere beyond me—not accessible through the drug—but the touch of Corbin's human hand brought some peace to my chaotic senses.

I stayed with the gentle, steady stroking, grateful for Corbin's willingness to comfort me, and grateful that I had been able to ask for her help.

Buddhism perceives existence as a vast interconnected whole, and one of the most beautiful and illuminating representations of this is the Net of Indra. Indra was one of the major deities of old India; Hua Yen Buddhism, developed in seventh-century China, provided the cosmic philosophical image of Indra's net to represent the organic interrelatedness of all existence. The net stretches through the universe, representing time in its vertical extension and space in its horizontal. In visualizing the net, one sees that at each point where the threads intersect, there is a crystal bead representing an individual existence. As Nancy Wilson Ross describes it, "Each one of these innumerable individual crystal beads reflects on its surface not only every other bead in the net but every reflection of every other bead, thus creating numberless, endless reflections of each other while forming one complete and total *whole*." Thus unity and multiplicity exist together, a vision that suggests that spiritual freedom is gained only in relationship with others.

This interpenetration of all phenomena is always stressed in Buddhism. I felt it particularly in the hospital, where I was surrounded by *sangha*.

Community (or *sangha* in Sanskrit) is one of the major dimensions of Buddhist engagement. We often think of Buddhist seekers as meditating alone in caves, in the forest, and on mountaintops for years at a time, so the emphasis on community may seem surprising; but the Buddha himself had stressed the importance of group allegiance and cooperation. Sitting in meditation by oneself and sitting in a roomful of people feel very different from each other. In a large room with others, I can feel my practice tangibly supported. Also, in a community, we are challenged to feel and act out the teachings in daily life. It is one thing to experience one's heart expand in compassion while meditating; it is another to keep an open mind and heart while dealing with an angry neighbor or coworker or partner.

In the hospital I felt the meaning of "sangha" grow and deepen, as I received the care of my Buddhist, feminist, political, theological, lesbian, neighborhood, and other friends, who came showing me the very purest part of themselves, whose motive was simply love. Included in that sangha were the nurses and aides who took care of me. I began to experience the net of human support that was forming around me, that would sustain me in the coming months.

The emphasis on community reminds us of our common experience. Along with all other creatures we share the elements that make up the world—earth, air, fire, and water—all this is what constitutes a human being. And we share a common trajectory: birth, coming to maturity, decline, and death. We are part of the great net that includes and reflects every being in the universe. So I surrendered to Corbin's hand on my back, and perhaps she felt my gratitude.

That evening, a small miracle occurred. A new batch of visitors had arrived. Loud violent cartoons blasted from the TV set, equipment clanged, and voices intruded—I felt as if my skin had been peeled away by the constant sensory assault. Behind the curtain, my roommate's visitors chattered.

Kathryn, a friend from the Graduate Theological Union, who sat beside my bed, must have sensed my distress, for she took my hand and began to hum the opening notes of "Amazing Grace." Her voice made a quiet stream under all the din.

Suddenly the TV set snapped off. Utter silence opened behind the curtain. Then several rich, deep female voices joined my friend's, and the gentlest, tenderest version of that venerable hymn rolled out to fill the room. *Amazing grace, how sweet the sound....*

Kathryn and I gazed in amazement at each other. My other two friends turned to stare at the curtain. The song went on, a heartfelt, holy rendering of this beautiful old hymn. I felt as though I were being rocked and held in nurturing arms.

When the last note sounded, Kathryn went to peer around the curtain. "That was so beautiful," she told the invisible singers. "We loved it."

In my scratchy post-surgery voice (impeded by the tube that ran down my throat to my stomach), I croaked out, "Could you do one more?"

They did. A precise, original rendition of "He Leadeth Me," a hymn I used to sing as a child in my Methodist Church in Ohio. I knew it well.

When the song finished, the atmosphere in the room had been transformed. We existed now in a comforting silence; and all the offending noises from the hallway sounded outside our bubble of peace. I felt myself smiling, relaxed for the first time since the surgery.

A beaming face looked around the curtain. "Hope you'll feel better soon," she said. I heard the women say a quiet goodnight to my roommate and walk out of the room.

The next day my roommate, Charlene, told me that the voices were those of her sisters, a singing group called the Webb Sisters. These three women had opened at the Monterey Blues Festival to a standing ovation and sang in African-American churches and religious gatherings regularly.

Yes, there were always rays of kindness or beauty available to me, if I could be present enough to receive them.

5

Help Me Make It through the Night

Healing hurts.
Nancy Berson

IN OUR LITTLE ROOM Charlene and I had come to know each other in a way: not the usual exchange of information, but of certain feelings. (I was to spend ten days in that room.) Charlene, who had diverticulitis, which would soon correct itself, frequently went downstairs to smoke a cigarette. (The patients stood in the cold air outside the lobby in their hospital gowns, puffing away.) Each time she dropped in on a particular patient friend. "Her husband got killed on the freeway," Charlene explained to me. "She couldn't accept it and she was grieving and just got to drinking, and it went on for so long her kidneys failed her. She's so messed up they can't do much for her."

Today when Charlene returned from her cigarette break, she looked stunned. Climbing into her bed in her hospital gown, she sat staring straight ahead, not even bothering to turn on the TV.

"How is she today?"

Charlene glanced sideways at me, with a look that said she was almost glad I was there.

"She passed."

We sat in silence until Charlene spoke again.

"When I went in the room, it was all cleaned out…no one in the bed. Then the nurse told me."

We sat looking at the beige wall. After ten minutes or so she roused herself and reached for the TV control. All afternoon, cartoons romped across the screen, and Charlene watched with distracted eyes, her face sullen and grieving.

Respecting her solitude, I pretended to read, but I could feel Charlene's shock and grief, and I thought of her friend so tragically broken. I wondered if there were something I could do to ease them both. So many times in the meditation hall at Dhamma Dena we had done the practice known as *metta,* or loving-kindness. In this we sent loving wishes—the classic formula was "May you be free from enmity. May you be free from grief and disease. May you be happy." Now, while I sat looking at the pages of my book, I opened my heart first to myself (for Buddhist compassion always begins with a gentleness toward oneself) and then I visualized Charlene in front of me and imagined her friend, whom I had never seen, with her. "May you be free from grief and suffering," I silently wished them. "May you find peace."

Three mornings after the operation the surgeon and residents found an infection developing in my wound. Half an hour later a doctor with crewcut hair arrived to lean over me and pull out most of the superficial staples in my belly as I gritted my teeth against the pain. He was a former navy doctor, scrubbed, brisk, new to the Highland environment. He assured me that the infection would heal now that the wound was open. When he had left the room, I lay shaken by the news. An infection! How bad was it? What might happen?

That night several friends came to visit me. Two of them were theater people, dramatically dressed in black and wearing extravagant pieces of jewelry. My navy doctor's eyebrows rose when he entered the room and saw them. He stood still for a moment, surprised, I presume, by my friends' relative vibrancy in this dreary environment.

Then he came to prod at the open wound in my belly, first pulling out the gauze pads, which stuck to the raw tissue. I groaned, and my friends' faces sharpened in sympathy.

The doctor poked at the wound with a Q-tip, and I lay gazing up at the top of his short black crewcut, astonished at the sensations of tearing and burning he was causing.

Peering worriedly at the doctor's busy hands, Naomi asked him what he thought about the prospects for the survival of Highland Hospital, given recent county budget cuts and the problems of America's rush to managed care.

"The place *ought* to be closed," he said, reaching for a fresh gauze pad. "The level of efficiency here is pretty low. They spend more money than other places to take care of people."

My friends stared at him, and I could feel them ruffling in annoyance.

"But what about the people who have no other recourse but Highland?" persisted Grace.

He leaned closer to my wound, talking over his shoulder at my friends, "You could take the money from here and give it to other hospitals where people would get better care."

"Do you *have* to put the gauze in there?" I asked him.

"Uh huh."

"Because then you'll have to pull it out again."

He lifted his head for the briefest glance into my eyes.

"Is it real bad?"

"It's bad enough."

He began stuffing the gauze inside my wound, its rough weave lacerating me.

"This is all for my own good, yes?" I asked.

"Believe it or not."

Straightening, he looked around at my friends with the expression of a man besieged. "What about getting more *funds* for the county?" Grace asked him. "Why can't the quality of care be improved!" said Naomi. For the first time he smiled, bemused by these mouthy women.

And then he was gone.

They took away my morphine, and the pain now made itself felt. All night I lay on my side, the tube in my nose rubbing against the tender tissue of the inside of my nostril. I held the tube with my hand, trying to position it so that it did not press into my flesh. The tube, attached to a humming machine, drained acids from my stomach out into a jar next to the bed. The acids that normally break down food would have burned through my stomach wall if they were not being pumped out by this machine, for no food came into my stomach now, and would not until the surgeons judged that the incision in my colon had sufficiently healed.

It was 1 A.M. Charlene's curtain was pulled, and she had turned off the TV set. From behind her curtain I heard faint snores.

I tried moving my shoulders up and down as I breathed deeply. The muscles of my back had cramped, aching dully. Carefully I turned in the bed, hoping to ease my lower back, to no avail. And with each movement the nose tube pulled against tissue already rubbed raw.

Worst of all was the pain in my belly. The open wound throbbed and burned under its gauze pads. To open up a belly, surgeons have to cut down through several layers of muscle. So to close it they have to suture successive levels, one at a time, from the deepest up to skin level. In my case, the top level was being kept open so that the infection could be treated. My navy doctor had assured me that the wound would eventually close by itself. The body would repair itself, pull skin surface to skin surface to knit them back together. How I hoped he was right.

I dozed, and woke to find it was only 2:30 A.M. Morning seemed impossibly distant, as I became aware again of the ache in my back, the pressure of the tube in my nostril. My hand smarted where the needle connecting me to the IV entered my skin.

To distract myself I looked at the bouquets and plants crowding my bed table. White mums in a pot, a bouquet of red roses; purple iris and delicate white baby's breath in a tall glass vase. Crystal's downstairs tenant had brought me a Halloween plant, held by a pumpkin-headed straw farmer figurine wearing a tall witch's hat. Cards stood among the plants and were taped to the walls. My sister had sent me a large cheerful get-well card from Florida.

Every evening my half of the room filled with visitors, and always among them was at least one Wandering Menstrual. They told me they had met at my house with Crystal and were setting up a schedule to care for me when I would be released. I was glad to see each person who came in the door, for they all arrived bringing love, concern, humor, and caring.

I was somewhat surprised by this generosity, particularly from people whom I did not know well. A student, a Zen master, a young woman who had gone to school with me at the Graduate Theological Union—arrived to sit with me, brought me gifts of audiotapes and books, a squeezable small rubber penguin (to counter anxiety), a precious smooth rock to hold.

The penguin stood on the bed table among the cards. I picked it up now and squeezed its soft, rubbery body, and soon drifted off again into sleep.

Later, waking, I found myself held down by a grid of pain. Here in the middle of this long night frustration rose in me, and I felt sorry for myself. Crystal had come to visit today, and we had talked about the upcoming performance of her choral work. I had gathered all my energy to help her find a way to work with the chorus members who had been resisting the challenging dissonances and multi-rhythms of her New Music composition. Entering with her into her dilemma, working with her to try to solve it, I felt some intimacy with her for the first time since our blow-up before the surgery. There was a sweetness to our encounter, Crystal overwhelmed by her responsibilities, I trying to give her useful ideas and calm her. No matter what else was happening between us, we had always been able to help each other with our work. But when she left, I lay exhausted, realizing that the conversation had drained me.

Now at three in the morning, as I stared up into the semi-darkness of the hospital room. My back throbbed, and the wound was fiery with pain.

What would Ruth Denison say about my dilemma? I summoned her to stand in her strong, square-shouldered body at the foot of my bed, her face inclined toward me. "Darling," I heard her say, "part of your pain is caused by your fear of the pain. You want so much for it to go away. You pull in the opposite direction, and so the pain grows bigger."

In many Dharma talks in the meditation hall at Dhamma Dena Ruth had discussed our fear and suffering.

"What if you were to surrender to it, to welcome it like a friend? You are very interested in your friend, you give all your attention to her. Can you give your attention to the pain? What are the sensations in your back? What is their nature, their intensity, their texture? Do they stay the same or do they change? Your pain is not so simple: it is a worthy object for your meditative inquiry. Can you be with it here? Can you return into this body/mind process and be faithful to it, investigate it, and see its insubstantiality?"

"All right, Ruth, all *right!*"

"Yes, darling, you try it. You know how to do it."

Slowly I pushed myself onto my side again, adjusted the tube in my nose, straightened the smaller tube from the needle in my hand to the hanging bag of fluids, and allowed myself to come as fully as I could into contact with my body. First I attended to my breath, watching as it slowed and deepened. Then I sent my consciousness to my lower back, where I found a thick hard girdle of sensations. I stayed there, watching this pain that seemed solid, being with it even though I felt the urge to escape. No, stay here. Be the observer.

Gradually, as I attended, the sensations in my back began to lose their solidity. Now I experienced movement, a pulse and flow, a chaotic dance of atoms. I could penetrate only so far, experiencing this agitation as my pain still, but I began to be genuinely interested in the nature of the sensations. Some of it hot, some like electrical currents twitching my nerves, some a flowing of particles. I held my consciousness there in my lower back, fascinated with the performance.

For a time the concentration steadied, even while part of my mind wanted to scream at the pain. From somewhere far away I heard a nurse's voice in the hallway. My roommate snorted, and turned in her bed. Still I stayed with the sensations in my back, focusing more and more fully into those tissues.

And finally there were only the sensations—without a name or a definition or association—only an elemental vibration of phenomena expressing life.

For a few moments I was able to stay with this experiencing of the flux in itself, separate from my identifications and desires. What a huge freedom it bestowed.

Then I fell back into my "I" and experienced the sensations as if they were attached to "me," and they became pain again. The tissues of my lower back complained loudly.

I spent the hours until dawn alternating between deep penetration into the sensations in the tissues and the energy there, and times of identifying and feeling this activity as "pain." Back and forth, engaged and then slipping away, engaging again.

Finally, light from the window came pale and thin into the room. I heard Charlene shift in her bed and I knew that soon the nurse would come.

Gradually the mechanical attachments that held me tied (like Gulliver to the ground) to a machine or an IV stand were removed. How to describe the relief when the nurse pulled out my nose-tube? True, it scraped the tissues excruciatingly as it came out, but then I could breathe unobstructed, both nostrils open. What joy my body felt.

And I drank some juice, for the first time in six days taking something into my mouth and swallowing it.

One afternoon Sandy Butler stood at the foot of my bed, radiating energy, her vitality making me aware of my own weakness. "Crystal sends her love," she told me. "She says she's so blitzed with her composing that she can't come today, but she's thinking of you." I imagined Crystal at the table where she wrote her music, her electric keyboard before her. For an instant my heart lurched with longing for her.

"How's the wound?" Sandy asked me.

"Um, sore."

"And when will you hear about the pathology report?"

Sandy was efficient as usual, but I couldn't help wondering how this felt to her, whether she was suffering emotional bleed-throughs from her partner's death. It had been during that difficult time that I had come to know Sandy. We had met earlier, in a feminist group, and I had been struck by her intelligence, her confidence, and her size; but I had made no effort to get to know her better. Then, when her partner was struggling with cancer, we became friends. Sandy would drive across the Bay Bridge from San Francisco, where she lived, to spend the afternoon with me in Oakland. Because I barely knew her partner and was not involved in her care I became an "outpost" for Sandy. We would walk under the trees in Mountain View Cemetery and talk of politics and literature, what was going on in the lives of Sandy's two grown daughters, what was happening in my life—anything but cancer and illness.

Sandy had walked fast and talked fast, doing her best to take a short respite from her sorrow as she told me about how thrilled she had been to deliver her first keynote address at a major conference, how she worked strongly and deeply with the women who staffed battered women's centers. Matching her stride for stride, I learned that Sandy loved jazz and knew a great deal about it. I realized that she cherished our visits because they reminded her that the world was larger than the context in which she watched her partner slowly losing her battle to live.

Now in Highland Hospital, in response to Sandy's question, I held up both my hands.

"What's wrong?" she asked.

"That's a hard subject."

"The pathology report?"

"Yeah."

Sandy dipped her head, looked at me for a moment above the rims of her glasses, and then came to sit down next to me on the bed. She put her arm around my shoulders. "I'm sorry I interrogated you like that."

Leaning back against her warm arm, I realized how much anxiety awoke in me when I thought of the pathology report. Somewhere in the great edifice of Highland Hospital a pathologist was slicing through the section of bowel they had removed from my belly, and cutting open the tumor. Another pathologist was bending over a microscope, examining the cells of the lymph nodes taken out with the bowel section, and speaking the words that a transcriptionist would type up—words that would determine my future.

Sandy and I sat in silence, her arm tight around me, and gazed out the window next to my bed at the bright autumn sky. Each day I saw the sky change from dawn to full sunlight to twilight. I watched the light play on the towers of the old hospital, built in Spanish mission style, with mud-red tile and creamy stucco. I had not been outside for seven days, had not felt the air on my skin or walked on earth or concrete. Desire consumed me: to escape into the outside world!

"It'll be another week before the path report is ready," I told Sandy. "Dr. Bold came to see me yesterday and told me to make an appointment to see him after I get out, so we can look at the report together."

"I'll go with you," she said, and then paused, "unless Crystal is going."

"Thank you," I told her.

When Sandy had gone, I listened to a tape of the Webb Sisters singing bluesy gospel, which Charlene had left me when she was released. The room felt so big without her. The tube through my nose must have irritated my throat because now I coughed. But with each cough my opened belly jerked, and pain shot through my torso. So I sipped from a glass of water and tried to quell the tickling in the back of my throat.

The wound in my belly was a long slit, open about an inch wide, pink and white inside. Dr. Bold and my navy doctor thought it looked great. But it hurt most all the time, and I asked for Tylenol.

My last night at the hospital, when all was still, I was awakened by running footsteps in the hallway. The male night nurse called out, "What's going on?" and a tight voice from the room next to mine demanded,

"Get suction!" I lay fully awake, hearing footsteps converge from all directions, voices, and a cart rolling down the hall, bumping the doorway as it careened into the next room. Someone's on the edge, I thought. They're reviving him. The noises went on for a while and then stopped, and one by one I heard the nurses leave the room. Ah, I thought, it's over. He's okay again, and slid into sleep.

That morning the view out the window looked so beautiful, with the light touching the trees and illuminating the little neat houses in a row across the street, making them appear as though they glowed from inside.

When Willa, the student nurse from Nigeria, came in to take my vital signs, I asked her about last night's uproar. She was a shy, very dark-skinned, hesitant person. She dipped her head. "He didn't make it."

"But why?"

"Nobody knows. We were checking his vital signs regularly, but when Rhonda went in to check him, he was already dead. We couldn't bring him back."

The man who died, she told me, had had back surgery. "But you don't die from that!" I objected.

She was leaning over my arm checking the IV needle that was still attached there. She straightened, and with two warm fingers touching my inner arm, she said, "Yes, but surgery itself—and the aftereffects—anything can happen." She paused, and then spoke again, in her lilting accent, "Respiration, and all of that—your system has been put into such an extreme state...."

When she left, I sat in the bed feeling in my body that somebody next to me had gone away. Willa had said the man was in his forties. I'm sure he had no idea, his family had no idea, that he would die from back surgery!

And here I sat, alive, waiting for my breakfast of "full liquids."

The "certified nurse assistant" came in with the breakfast tray. She was from Africa or the Caribbean—I couldn't tell which from her accent. This morning she did not look at me as she slammed the tray down. I saw that she had brought the wrong items. "Excuse me," I said, "I'm supposed to have full liquids, not clear liquids." Her eyes rolled and she jerked her shoulders. "This *is* full liquids!" she snapped, and turned to flounce out of the room. I felt as though she had slapped me.

From the hallway I heard her loud irritated voice, and then someone else objecting, "She's insulting me!" Then a chaos of voices erupted, the nurse assistant delivering a scathing commentary on everyone's character defects that I could barely understand through her juicy accent, while several other voices matched her volume, ranting at her. Finally she threatened, in a raspy growl, "*I'll tear your throat out!*"

I sat up straighter in bed, my nerves tingling awake in response to the incipient violence, while my mind searched for a story. What could have sent this woman over the edge—the man's dying last night? a fight with her husband?—for she sounded utterly out of control. Now I heard the nurses talking her down, gently reprimanding her, soothingly hushing her.

Her words stayed in my mind. "I'll tear your throat out!" What a magnificent threat. Would she do it with her teeth, with her fingernails? I lay back again, enjoying the drama, feeling my mood improve.

Except that I realized I now had the problem of getting a breakfast of full liquids.

I thought again of the man who had died next door. My body too had been put into "such an extreme state," balanced tenuously between life and death so they could cut me open and reach inside. I had teetered on that edge and had fallen over on the side of life, but I could as easily have fallen into death. "It is the nature of all things that take form to dissolve again," the Buddha said.

I felt the tears begin to pool at my eyes and then brim over, spilling down my cheeks. Tears fell on my hands, on my hospital gown. I felt a great sad relief for myself, and a deeper sadness for the man who had died and his family. I cried for my trauma and my pain, and for his. And I felt sorry for the certified nurse assistant hysterical with rage: what terrible thing could have happened to her to provoke that?

Tears flowed down my face, and I began to gasp and sob. I let it go on, not trying to cry, not trying to stop crying, just letting the tears fall onto my hands, my rumpled gown.

"Oh, what is wrong?"

I glanced sideways to see Willa in the doorway, holding a breakfast tray, her eyes in her kind face round with concern.

"It's okay," I choked out. "I'm really okay."

She put down the tray and then lingered next to my bed. I wanted her to leave so I could be alone with my sorrow and relief. And soon she did.

PART TWO

6

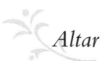

Altar

*Everybody has a mind that can expand. But you have to
cultivate that kind of mind. Now comes the letting go
of obstructions, the stretching of the mind towards
the impossible, towards that which says,
"there is nothing left except peace."*

Ayya Khema

IN THE LIVING ROOM, inside a tall rough-wood hutch, I had gathered candles, incense, stones, and a sea shell to form an altar. When I came home
from the hospital, I began to add to it photographs of people dear to me
who had died. I wanted to commune with those who existed now in
another condition. Zen master Maurine Stuart looked out at me from a
resolute face, one eyebrow raised, eyes challenging me to "not make a
move to avoid" whatever came my way. After that first glimpse of her at
the Women and Buddhism conference, I had learned more about her.
Head of the Cambridge Buddhist Association for many years, Maurine
had been a concert pianist, a mother, and wife. She embodied the powerful Zen presence, that capacity to be completely there with you in this
moment. She was utterly a Zen master, and also utterly a wife and mother, an artist, a woman. She was greatly loved. She had died of cancer some
years before, but I still felt her presence, as vibrant as it had been on that
first day I saw her at the conference, impressive in her black robe, and on
other days when I had visited her in her Cambridge apartment and listened as she played Bach and Beethoven, or sat drinking tea with her in
her kitchen.

Taped to the doors of the hutch were photographs of Tibetan altars in
Dharamsala, India. There a Western woman, a friend of someone who

knew me, had arranged for healing prayers to be recited for me by the lamas. She wrote, "In Bodhanath [a Buddhist temple], twice now I have made offerings on your behalf for ceremonies of healing and overcoming obstacles." The photographs showed colorful constructions of scarves and gods' eyes surrounded by butter lamps and *tormas,* ritual offerings that looked like lumpy candles. She had prevailed upon a lama, in his pilgrimage to the holy city of Bodhgaya, the site of the Buddha's enlightenment, to offer flowers, lamps, and incense on my behalf. I knew that people here were praying for me as well.

From a strict Theravada Buddhist perspective, which eschews deities, the concept of prayer would make no sense; but my involvement with the goddess Kwan Yin had opened me to the concept of participation by other dimensions of reality in the events of ordinary life. Like meditation, prayer in Buddhism can be a way of connecting us with the ultimate deep nature of the universe. Through prayer, we become receptive to a more spacious consciousness, tapping into the love and compassion available for all beings.

Dr. Larry Dossey, a medical researcher, had demonstrated that prayer affects healing, whether the patient knows she is being prayed for or not. Dossey showed that distance does not weaken the effect of the prayer, so the chanting of Tibetan men in maroon robes halfway across the world might actually affect me. If "reality...is non-local," then the world might be filled with innumerable influences coming from many locations and underlying the events of my daily life.

I would need all the help I could get, for I had gone several days before to hear the results of the pathology report. In the noisy surgery clinic, I was accompanied by neither Crystal nor Sandy, but a friend from the Graduate Theological Union named Victoria. With her at my side, I sat knee to knee with Dr. Bold, who showed me the blurry copy of the report and told me what they had discovered in surgery: the cancer had grown into the wall of my colon. And then the worst of the news. "Two of twenty-seven lymph nodes positive—that means the tumor had already spread to two lymph nodes." Victoria put a steadying hand on my shoulder. "Now I'm going to draw," Dr. Bold said. "I think you saw one of my drawings before so you already know what a lousy artist I am." He outlined a long curved tube. "That's your colon, kind of like a question mark: little appendix hangs off here, and your small intestine is in the middle. Your tumor was over here, we took it out. We felt the liver, felt all over, and we didn't find any other source of tumor. And when we do the operation we take out all the lymph nodes too. A couple of cells had gotten loose and were in those lymph nodes."

Dr. Bold paused and looked up from his drawing.

"So that's not so good," I said. "That's Stage Three, right?"

"Yes." He nodded. "But there's something we can do about it. For people who have a risk of the cancer growing somewhere else, but so small that we can't see it using X-rays or looking at it at the time of operation…we can do something to decrease the risk that the tumor will come back. For colon cancer, we use chemotherapy."

At home, sitting before my altar, careful of my still-open surgery incision, I looked at the picture of Lex Hixon, a distinguished scholar of religion and initiated master in a number of traditions. I remembered first seeing him in an auditorium in San Francisco, where he was to present poems from his book *Mother of the Universe*. Lex explained that a dancer would first come onto the stage, but we were to understand that she had been transformed from an ordinary woman into the goddess Kali, embodiment of the original energy that creates all life, and destroys it too. Kali is a wrathful goddess, and yet represents the maternal, for in a profound way life and birth are bound up with death and destruction. Kali is Creatrix, Protector, and Destroyer all in one. Lex was asking us to imagine that the goddess would literally arrive in the body of the dancer.

When a small woman in a scarlet sari entered the stage, a shiver went through the audience. What were we seeing? And then, in a gesture so unknown to us and so complete in itself that we gasped, Lex, a large-bodied, bearded man, got down on his knees and then lowered himself into a full prostration at the dancer's bangled feet. In that gesture of utter surrender, he revealed her as the goddess herself. Some women began to weep; I felt my breath stop in my chest.

Later I had spoken to Lex, who held my hand as we talked, and I thought, "If I were ever going to study with a scholar, it would be this one." I had even considered moving temporarily to the East Coast, where Lex lived, to become his student.

Now that the cancer was here in me, Lex arrived in a meditation. In a dark woodland clearing he stood, lumbering, bear-like. I could see that where his heart should have been, a lavender crystal rose glowed in his chest, radiating light. I desperately wanted to have such a luminous flower in my own chest. In answer to my plea Lex said, "If you can stay strong for this whole year, you can have a heart like this."

In the bleak, curtained cubicle at the hospital Dr. Bold explained, "Your tumor had already gotten to the point where cells were breaking loose from the tumor itself. The job of the lymph nodes is to catch everything that gets away. So they were doing their job and picked up some cells, but we don't know for sure if maybe one cell got through and hadn't been picked up. Or two cells."

Victoria asked, "So if it's out there floating around in the blood vessels at this point, where is it going to land?"

"The liver is the most likely place. It's still cancer of the colon, but it's called metastatic or spread-to-the-liver. It's just cancer of the colon that's growing in the liver. The best chance of taking care of it is when the cells are few in number; it's always easier when you're killing ten rather than a hundred billion cells. That's why we would say that it's better to treat you without knowing for sure if you have it and give you all the benefit of curing you when those cells are few in number, rather than ignoring the possibility that a couple of cells have started growing in your liver and waiting five or seven years and *then* trying to treat you. That's just a recommendation. I want you to meet with our oncologists too, and they can give you some more information."

"Couldn't we just keep track of it? Do tests every six months or something?" I asked.

"The way we would look to see if it's growing in your liver is to do blood tests," Dr. Bold said, "but the thing is, if it gets to the point where we could detect any abnormalities on your blood test, that would mean it was already pretty advanced." He paused. "Roughly thirty to forty percent of people in your situation have cells spread to other locations. On the other hand, sixty to seventy percent never have colon cancer again."

I stared at Dr. Bold as he explained that the oncologist would probably recommend the standard protocol of forty-eight weeks of weekly infusions of chemicals. Forty-eight weeks! I couldn't imagine it.

Lex Hixon had died a few weeks after my surgery of colon cancer, which was caught at a too-advanced stage to be helped. As a young man he had written:

I simply assert
that all is light:
the sea, the hills, the horses, the symphonies....
all I want
inscribed on the dancing flames of my pyre:
the enigmatic phrase,
all is light.

Now I had cause to think of death, to imagine an errant cancer cell making its way through my belly toward my liver, where it would enter that juicy organ and begin to divide, piling up cells into tissue to become a mass, a lump, a little monster more deadly than the last.

And so I looked at the faces of the dead and thought about the Buddhist description of the self. Zen master Joko Beck (happily, still alive) describes a stream in which small whirlpools form. They have a shape, they gather debris, and swirl around for a time, still part of the stream and the water yet distinguished from it; and then a rock shifts on the bottom, the whirlpool dissolves, the debris floats away, and there is nothing but the flow again. So we are, each of us, an arrangement of energy that holds together for a time and then breaks apart, dissolves, and returns into the flow.

When a student asked Joko if she meant that life was no different from death, she replied, "There is no life and death, *and* there is life and death. When we know only the latter, we cling to life and fear death. When we see both, the sting of death is largely mitigated." The whirlpool and the water, relative and absolute reality—sitting here in life talking to the dead, I was contemplating both.

When we left Dr. Bold and came out of the hospital, Victoria took my arm. "How are you? Do you think you're capable of driving?" because we had foolishly come in separate cars. I took stock, feeling not quite present, not fully in my body. "Let's sit down here," she urged. We sat on a low brick wall. Victoria, a theology student and theatrical director, seemed to know exactly how to help. "Now put both your feet flat on the ground," she told me. I did that, feeling its hardness under my shoes. We sat in silence, and I welcomed the autumn sun on my face. "You don't have to decide now," Victoria said. "We'll hear what the oncologist has to say. Give yourself time to look into it. Dr. Bold said you should take a month to recover from the surgery before you start the chemo, so you have a month to do some research." I nodded, gazing across the street at the neat small houses with their stucco facades, painted steps, and small mowed lawns. Gradually the houses settled from an expanded floating presence into their normal contours. I began to be aware of my breath, and sitting there, I followed it in and out, in and out, returning gratefully into my wounded, threatened body.

On my altar at home sat a photograph I took of my mom and dad some months before his death. I had gone with her to the nursing home to visit him. We had wheeled him in his wheelchair out into the garden, and she had pulled up a chair to sit next to him. They leaned together with their heads touching, his arm around her shoulder and her hand on his. He was eighty-two, she seventy-nine, the love between them still strong. When I was growing up, I had watched my Dad kiss my Mom goodbye each morning before he went off to work, and in the afternoon when he came home in his sweat-stained white carpenter's overalls, once again he greeted her by gathering her in his arms. He was always telling us how beautiful she was, what a wonderful figure she had, pointing out her creamy skin and the beauty of her dark-red wavy hair, and my mom, who was shy, would blush and urge him to stop.

We lived in the scruffy outskirts of Columbus, in a white frame house that barely contained the five of us. We did not have a television set until I was thirteen years old. Then, in the evening, Mom and Dad would sometimes lie on the couch together, arms around each other, watching Milton Berle or Midwestern Hayride; sometimes they sat in their separate chairs—hers with a straight back and flowered upholstery, his a huge green plastic contour chair—and read the newspapers, smoking cigarettes and commenting to each other now and then on the day's events.

I had a special relationship with my daddy, begun when I was a very young child. In the hot Ohio summer, I stroked the black curls of his chest hair as I leaned against his warm brown skin, my ear to his chest. I could feel his solidness, dense flesh, and sense the big bones of his rib cage like antlers curved around his heart. My daddy's head above mine looked out across the muddy creek where my brother and sister splashed and screamed. When he spoke, the vibration entered my ear, a furry buzzing. His body attended to me, holding me on his lap. Half asleep, I moved my foot drowsily on his brown knees that were laced with hair. He was speaking to Mom; through half-open eyes I saw her pale blue dress, her freckled hand, and the gold ring on her finger. We three sat in the shade; I was too young to join my siblings in the brown creek water. My daddy had taken me, earlier, and dipped me, his hands so big they completely encircled my chest.

Now as he held me I was almost asleep, surrendered, utterly safe; he would never drop me, no harm could come. I drank this luxury; warm and somnolent I drifted, gazing from the shade out into sunlight, listening to the wild shouts from the creek, until they faded and it was only the steady bump, bump, bump of my daddy's heart that I knew, and the safe big enclosure of his body.

As I grew up and my brother refused to spend time with him, I became my father's companion on fishing forays, in long days of yard or garden work. My daddy taught me to work, and praised me for doing it. One day at the age of twelve or so, while on a ladder pushing a paint roller across the living room ceiling, I looked down to see my dad watching me proudly. Turning to my mother, he said, "She's a good worker." Highest praise. He became a small contractor, building one modest house at a time, lavishing care on each detail; he mortgaged the house we lived in to finance these endeavors, risking our security—and each time was able to sell the newly built house before the next loan payment was due. We ate lots of potatoes and spaghetti; my mother sewed most of our clothes and combed the stores for bargains. But my father was able to build the houses he designed himself, and that, we understood, was better than a paycheck from some big construction company. It was worth the sacrifice. From watching him I learned that one could take risks, and disaster would not follow.

Ultimately my father and I entered a long conflict, as he criticized my life-choices—my politics, my hairdo, and my friends; and as soon as I was able to be on my own I fled Ohio and my family. But I always loved him best.

Next to the picture of my parents I had propped a photograph of my brother George, with his handsome face, crisp dark hair, his brown eyes shining. My only, precious brother could never please my father: they always fought, and my father always won. George grew up withdrawn and hesitant, and at the age of twenty-eight he put a pistol to his head and pulled the trigger. I had been nineteen years old, plunged without warning into that violence, followed by that huge absence. Forty-five years had not blurred the circumstances of his death, which had sent me into a distorted and dangerous period in my own life.

Now, faced with what could be my own death, I had a dream in which George and I sat naked, back to back, our hands clasped, connected to each other by a shared cowl of blood vessels. I understood that he would accompany me on this cancer journey, holding the experience in some other dimension while I lived it in this one.

I reached to touch the photograph, and with his face in my mind I closed my eyes and focused on my breath, sinking soon into concentration.

When I was newly home from the hospital, I had had to stay in bed and could not cook or care for myself. Crystal, in the midst of her composing, had interrupted her work to spend many hours on the phone and to greet the people who came bringing meals or just to visit. When we had come into our bedroom together for the first time in ten days, I found on the pillow a beautiful, hand-lettered card in Crystal's curvy script reading, "Welcome Home, Sweetheart," and on the bedstand rested a bouquet of purple flowers from the garden. She tucked me gently into the bed and pulled the blankets up. "I'm so glad you're home," she said, leaning to kiss my cheek.

But the demands of organizing my care while working to finish her commission had pushed her to the edge of her strength and sanity. She stayed up most of the night in her study, came to bed so wired she could barely sleep, and had to get up earlier than she wanted to start again. Even though she slept in the bed next to me, it seemed that I saw her only in passing, as she brought someone into the room to visit me, as she leaned in to tell me she loved me before disappearing into her studio. I was glad that Crystal was continuing her work even in this difficult situation, and I vowed to get well enough to go to the performance, which was a month from then.

As I grew stronger, I knew it was time to decide about the chemotherapy. Sandy Butler went to Planetree Health Resource Center in San Francisco and returned with reports of thirty trials of chemotherapy for colon cancer. Sitting next to each other on the couch in my living room, Sandy and I read the many pages of medicalese and absorbed the statistics. In the groups of patients studied, the recurrence rate without treatment was fifty percent; with treatment the recurrence rate dropped to twenty-five percent. Those numbers I found compelling. When I imagined discovering in a year that I had liver cancer, and thinking, "I wonder if chemotherapy would have prevented this," I decided to accept the treatment.

But I hated the thought of putting poison into my system, of risking the toxic side effects.

In mid-November I composed a letter to all the people who had expressed concern for me. The day I sent it I had read in *Turning Wheel*, the journal of the Buddhist Peace Fellowship, "I glimpse the limitless world of wholeheartedness, where one fate is lashed to that of all...." and it seemed that I too was glimpsing that way of living. I thanked my friends, and then told them my plan.

I have decided to undergo the course of chemotherapy they've suggested. It was not an easy decision.

The chemo I'll receive is a "mild dosage," according to the oncologist, who assures me it will not cause me to lose my hair or make me deathly ill. It may cause me considerable fatigue.

Before the beginning of this treatment, I will be doing everything possible to build up my immune system so that I can tolerate the chemo well. My acupuncturist is consulting with a practitioner who has worked in Chinese hospitals, where chemotherapy is coordinated with a program of acupuncture and herbs to support the immune system, which we will follow. I will be eating a cleansing diet. I am already taking an herbal preparation called Essiac, which is known to inhibit, even cure, cancer. I will be working with visualizations and meditation. First I need to recover from the surgery, then to build up my system for that first very intense five-day dose of chemo.

For a year I'm going to be spending substantial time at Highland Hospital. I have met the two oncology nurses, and both are exemplary human beings. I trust they will help me through this.

It's going to be rough for a while here at home. I'm still recuperating from the operation and not able to start my classes or other work yet. After only a few hours of being in the world, I have to lie down again. At the end of this month the chemo will begin, and that will be another challenge to my energy and state of mind. I doubt that I will be able to get back to my full work schedule until the beginning of the year.

But a dimension of this experience that has been heartening and healing is the support from you in my several communities: the Buddhist community, the feminist and lesbian communities, my Wandering Menstruals group, the Center for Women and Religion community of women with whom I went to China to the NGO Forum, my writing students, my women's spirituality sisters, my artist sisters, all my dear old friends who have known me for some of the thirty-five years that I have lived in the Bay Area, and new friends like the kind folks at Monte Vista Market. Your presence in my life is so supportive and healing.

One friend said to me, "There's really no need to thank anyone. This isn't extraordinary, this is just what we as a community of conscious women (and a few men) do when someone needs help." Well, maybe. But I want to thank every one of you who's held me in your thoughts and wished me well, who's made a gift of time, or food, or a prayer, an errand, whatever; you show me in a real, tangible way that we're in this life together, sharing ourselves wholeheartedly, with boundless courage. I love you.

7

At Land's End

*From the very beginning, there's nothing wrong.
There's no separation: it's all one radiant whole.*

Joko Beck

IN EARLY OCTOBER, a week before I was diagnosed with cancer, a fire
had erupted in Point Reyes National Seashore. This spit of land is shaped
roughly like the head of a coyote, its long snout poking into the Pacific.
Point Reyes comprises a hundred square miles of meadow, woodland, and
beach along the California coast.

Since coming to California so many years ago, I had loved to drive out
to Point Reyes, walk its beaches, lie in the tall dunes, and look out from
the cliffs over the ocean. Crystal and I came often on Sundays to ride
bicycles out the trails to the sea, or hike in to a lagoon and bird sanctuary behind the beach. On our way to the ocean we could see Douglas fir
and Bishop pine forests, live oaks, and California laurels; harbor seals lolled
on some of the beaches, and always birds flew overhead: gulls and spar-
rows, marsh hawks, kites, and red-tailed hawks. After a day spent in the
brisk ocean air we would stop in the little town of Point Reyes Station
for dinner, and drive home tired and sated with the vast comforting presence of land and water.

Fire raged at Point Reyes. On the nightly news, we watched smoke
billow above orange flames as the fire ate up thousands of acres of park-
land. We saw the crumbling black shells of the houses destroyed in the
tiny town of Inverness. The chaparral ridges and California-laurel valleys
around Limantour Road stood black, bare and smoking.

It was only a few days after the fire when I discovered I had cancer,
and felt the destruction wrought by the flames with a special harshness.

Now, on a Sunday in early December, I read that the ravaged seashore had begun to show signs of life returning. The idea gripped me. I had begun the chemotherapy with five straight days of treatment, and the 5FU and Levamisole had hit my body hard. The oncologist's saying that I might "feel tired" became a joke: I was exhausted, and had almost completely lost my appetite. All manner of food tasted the same to me—bland and nauseating. The inside of my mouth felt burned and raw with sores; and sores had also formed in my esophagus, so that food and drink went partway down, then seemed to hit a snag and hurt terribly. In order to eat, I was having to first dribble a liquid anesthetic down my throat. The chemicals put in to kill the cancer were destroying all the fast-dividing cells of my body, not discriminating between malignant cells and those of my mucous membranes.

That Sunday, although I drooped with fatigue, I desperately wanted to drive with Crystal out to Point Reyes to see the grasses and ferns poking up on the blackened hillsides, the sprouting bushes pushing green shoots up through the ashes—evidence that life had survived the devastation. Now that Crystal's performance was over, she had more time, and we were planning to go after she finished some chores outside.

I sat at the kitchen table, trying to swallow small bites of toast, when Crystal came up the back steps from the yard. Her face looked strange, blue eyes squinted, mouth hard. She began to talk about the money I owed her and my responsibilities in the house. Her words came in a relentless torrent, as if she had been talking to herself out in the yard, working up her fury, and now was pouring it out on me.

I sat, bent over, listening as Crystal paced and talked, stopped to press her hands on the tabletop and glare at me, then paced some more. I tried to answer her, but her words filled the kitchen, driving out everything but her rage.

Some of what Crystal was saying was the truth. I had not been an equal partner in the house, since I had no interest in owning a house and was not financially able to put anything down on it. I had paid off some of her loan to me and then had not been consistent with payments: she was absolutely right about that, and in that sense I had been disrespectful of her, scrupulously repaying any small debt I owed someone else while slacking off on my debt to her. The worst betrayal had been my raising money to go to China while neglecting to repay the money that

I owed her. Yet, given my condition right now, the idea that I could work more in the house and pay more money did not seem feasible. Crystal must know this: I wondered if her outburst came from fear—that I might die and leave her. Maybe there would be a way for her to get some help with her fears; I knew that there were support groups for the partners of cancer patients.

"Absolutely not!" she replied when I broached this. Her eyes blazed at me. "This is *not* about *something deeper*,"—her lip curled—"it is only about the money you owe me and the way you take advantage of me!"

Suddenly I found myself struggling to hold back tears. My chest felt carved out and hollow, hurting as much as my throat when I tried to swallow. I had no idea how to make the situation better. Wistfully I thought of the seashore and the tiny green plants waking up in that burned-out environment. I wished I could see them, and show them to Crystal. Maybe we could still escape the city, go together out into the sea air, relax and come to some balance with each other.

"No," she said, with vehemence, "we should be separate today!"

I went to find my jacket and put on my shoes. As I left the house, Crystal did not look up from the stacks of business papers she had spread across the kitchen table.

For a few minutes I sat in the car in the driveway. The firestorm of Crystal's fury had shaken me. I felt how vulnerable I was, without energy, and knew I could not stand up to her. As I had when Crystal had insisted that I get life insurance, I felt attacked. Apparently she had been harboring these complaints against me for years. Had she been so intimidated by me that she was afraid to bring up her concerns? It was true that I was, in normal life, a large energetic person, true also that I sometimes got angry at Crystal and even yelled at her. And I resisted talking about money. Had my behavior so frightened her that she could not speak to me about her dissatisfaction? Or was it a pattern we had both created, of not addressing the problems between us but simply living along on the surface?

I leaned my head against the steering wheel, overwhelmed by these questions, and realized that I did not have the strength to reach inside to a loving understanding of Crystal or to see her just now as my friend and partner who also needed help. My compassion failed me; I only felt her rage at me weighing like a great black blanket thrown over my head, stopping my breath. I had to escape it. Somehow I would make my way out to Point Reyes to see the tangible proof of new life emerging.

I turned the ignition key, felt the motor kick in, and pulled out from our driveway.

Driving through the streets of Oakland took all my concentration. I wondered if I would be able to handle the freeway.

On the radio, I heard a program about AIDS, and listened hungrily, comforted that others were suffering too. Now I had to enter the freeway. I talked to myself, "You are driving. Stay focused right here." Briefly I imagined losing control, crashing the car, and knew I would do everything I could to prevent that. I heard Ruth Denison's voice as she spoke to us of the "driving meditation" she always did. She had sat in the meditation hall before us, pretending to hold a steering wheel in her hands, and had demonstrated how to bring one's attention to all the many complicated dimensions of the experience of driving a car, to make ourselves conscious of the activity rather than losing ourselves in thoughts and fantasies. Now I applied her method, bringing my awareness to my hands on the steering wheel, to the pressure of my foot on the accelerator, to my view of Route 80 with its river of cars. I said to myself, "Driving, driving" as I crossed the Richmond Bridge, continually reminding myself what I was doing. "I am driving. Right now I am driving." I gathered my mind into this task.

As I approached the green hills of Marin, a great wave of fatigue washed over me. Despite myself, I imagined how it would have been if Crystal had been with me, sharing the anticipation. But I was driving, I reminded myself, and gathered my strength once again, giving all my attention to the moving car, the road before me.

I entered the little town of Fairfax and saw the familiar landmarks— Spanky's restaurant, the Siam Lotus Thai restaurant. Across from Spanky's was the coffeehouse where Crystal and I always stopped on our way out. Sometimes we sat at a little table and sipped lattes and talked, before going on. The memory brought pain. How I missed the softness and caring that we had shared at first. It came only in moments now—with a card or a flower, an apology, a wish for me—and then was gone, as if her hurt and disappointment had sent her to live in a castle completely shut away from me; now and then she reached out of a window to touch me, but then quickly withdrew her hand.

Leaving Fairfax I drove out through densely wooded, rolling hills. The ocean seemed a very great distance away. Again I focused on what I was doing, "Driving," I reminded myself, leaving other thoughts behind. A meadow with black and white cows peacefully grazing opened out to my right.

At Woodacre I saw the sign for Spirit Rock Meditation Center, the driveway curving out past a fenced lot where horses stood, and hills climbed up in rounded contours against the cloudy sky. I had come often to this place to hear Buddhist teachers, to participate in sittings or celebrations. I thought again of how easy it was to sit in a meditation hall and feel loving-kindness in oneself for every living creature; how hard it is to practice that in daily life, when we struggle to protect ourselves from our own and others' anger. I felt my failure to move beyond my self-protectiveness and see into Crystal's heart. She, my closest person, had become mysterious and threatening to me.

Soon the trees drew closer down to the road, reaching across it with feathered branches, and I saw the straight red-brown trunks of redwoods and the mass of smaller trees crowding in among them. Tucked in here and there in the deep shade stood brown shingle houses.

Entering under the stately trees of Samuel P. Taylor Park, I rolled down my window. The chemo had stolen my sense of smell, but I could remember that fresh pungency of trees wet from a recent drizzling rain. In the park the trees grew even thicker, and a stream ran beside the road, plashing over rocks and fallen branches.

Then the trees fell away, and a rocky hillside with brown and black cows appeared on my right. The sky seemed huge above them. Among the hills, the aluminum roofs of barns reflected the weak light. I was coming to the top of a hill. With great relief, I found myself rolling down the slope toward Olema. I could stop for a rest. In the Olema Farm House restaurant, I sat at a small table and ordered a bowl of clam chowder and a piece of warm crusty French bread. Then I went to the restroom, took out my little bottle of anesthetic, and with the eyedropper sent some of it down my throat. I was able to eat the soup and bread, chewing and swallowing carefully, able to tolerate the scraping of the food against my tissues, though I tasted nothing but a slight sour edge of wine in the soup.

Driving out again on the curvy road to Limantour, the road climbed up, a narrow winding strip, and I saw moss on the trees. Now dizzy with fatigue, I saw no evidence of the fire. Could this be the wrong place—hadn't the paper said Limantour? Should I turn around and go back?

But then I began to see the blackened trunks of trees near the road and stretches of bare black ground where the undergrowth had been devastated. And gradually the trees and brush gave way to a wasteland—hill after hill covered with a scrim of black-gray ash and nothing else, here and there a lone skeleton of a tree still standing.

Suddenly I crested a hill and over misty heights could see out to the ocean, but I could not make out the actual shore. The charred hills seemed to spread all the way to the water, and looking at them, I began to wonder about the animals who had lived here. What had happened to the deer, foxes, and bobcats, the coyotes and raccoons? The owls! The butterflies! I drove through this devastated landscape in horror. Then I remembered to look for the new shoots, and caught sight of a few sprays of green standing up defiantly from the ashes. Yes, here they were: life returning.

As I neared the ocean, still the burned hills went on, and now I could see the estero behind the beach, an old valley that had been filled by the sea and was now separated from the surf by great sand bars. Light reflected off the water, making the estero appear as a long silver strip laid against the dark land. Beyond rose the dunes and the great shifting waves of the Pacific.

I came down the last hill and saw that the fire had in fact eaten all the way to the sea. The thick underbrush of the bird sanctuary was gone, leaving only a charred strip of ground next to the water. What had happened to the birds, to their nests, the insects they feed on?

I parked in the lot and got out, but had only enough strength to walk to the edge of the gravel and look out across the estero and the stripped land. I stood with the sea wind in my face, feeling a deep weariness in every part of my body.

When I returned to the car, I rested my head on the back of the seat, and dreaded the drive back to town. No, I told myself, stay here. But this landscape of death was so painful. I closed my eyes, breathed in, breathed out. I thought of *tonglen*, the Tibetan Buddhist practice of transforming negativity. This is a technique of giving and receiving that allows us to approach the suffering we see around us and be with it, rather than pulling away and hardening our hearts to protect ourselves. *Tonglen* begins by drawing in the suffering, hatred, or destruction with our in-breath, as though it were a cloud of oily black smoke. This dark cloud enters us and penetrates to the core of our being, where it loosens our preoccupation with self. Then we exhale, sending out a cooling light, with wishes for joy and well-being. We give the best of ourselves for the healing of the world. From this general beginning we can move to particular beings or situations of suffering, and work to transform that pain first in ourselves and then in others.

I decided to try the practice and I breathed in terror—taking into myself the fear the animals must have experienced as they raced to escape the fire, that of the birds as they fluttered through the smoke away from their burning nests—and with my outbreath I sent them a wish for peace and comfort, wherever they were now. I breathed in anger—my own anger that this destruction had happened, Crystal's rage at me, and the fury of everyone in the world who is hurt and scared—and as I breathed out I wished us all surrender and tranquillity. I breathed in weariness—the deep exhaustion of all those who must work too hard just to survive, those who were ill like me, and those weary unto death—and in my outbreath I sent strength, steadiness, and faith in what is.

In and out I breathed, pulling in pain that was dark and heavy like this landscape. I breathed in for every suffering creature in the universe, willing now to let this pain enter me deeply. And then I gave back all the goodness and enjoyment, humor, and faith in life I had ever felt. In and out, in and out.

When I opened my eyes, I felt a growing sense of peace.

I sat looking out at the gray moving surface of the ocean, and a song began in my mind. It was a chant to Yemaya, the Yoruba goddess of the ocean and creator of all life, that I had learned years ago from the singing group Alive! *Ye ye ye Yemaya, Yemaya....* In the newspaper, a park ecologist had described the long-term benefits of the fire. It had melted the resin off the Bishop pine tree cones, releasing the seeds onto the ground and creating the beginnings of whole new forests. Because of the ash, the nutritional quality of the vegetation would increase, and thus the animals and birds would benefit from a richer diet. As I looked around here now, it was hard to imagine it green again, but I knew that the few infant sprays I had seen would guarantee that.

Always the lessons of impermanence surround us. The Buddhist teaching that the phenomenal world moves in a never-ending flow of matter and energy is nowhere more obvious than at the ocean's edge. The very piece of land on which I sat was moving, inch by inch, up the California coast. The narrow wedge of rock now called Point Reyes had started three hundred miles to the south at Los Angeles millions of years ago, and continued to travel north. The beaches constantly changed, cliffs eroding, and sand shifting. My body was healing; the wound in my belly was almost closed, even as the chemo dragged me down. The land would heal from the fire, and another fire would come, or an earthquake would rip the surface of the land apart.

Nothing solid; nothing to hold onto but the inevitability of change.

I sat in my car watching the sky darken above the sea, knowing I would soon have to drive home to Oakland and return to face Crystal. I breathed in and out, connected once again to the sensations of my body. "Breathe, and know that you are alive," Ruth Denison would slowly intone. "Breathe, and know that all is helping you. Breathe, and know that you are the world." Feeling the air enter my nostrils, I sensed how much I was a part of this great shifting landscape of earth and water. I watched as a gull banked on the wind above the car, showing me the white flash of its under-wings as it hovered. Then it swooped away, and I breathed out. Comforted, for a moment.

8

Knitting Time, 1984

The spiritual journey involves going beyond hope and fear,
stepping into unknown territory, continually moving forward.
Pema Chodron

AT DHAMMA DENA, during the meditation retreats, insight was encouraged in many dimensions. The silence opened around me, offering possibilities for new ways of experiencing myself and others; the desert itself, with its plants so delicately adapted for life in this harsh environment, its birds and snakes, rabbits and insects, its towering sky and distant mountains, taught myriad lessons about impermanence and the preciousness of all life. Ruth offered various kinds of practices, from formal sitting and walking meditation to improvised slow movement sessions and fast-paced walks across the desert; she showed us how to be mindful while eating, while working; sometimes she would have us march to music or dance to drums, or sit in silence listening as she rang a set of hanging bells at the front of the meditation hall; she spontaneously created small rituals and ceremonies for us to perform: she was bent upon showing us how to be mindful in every moment of our lives.

In her "Dharma talks," Ruth presented the great truths of Buddhism and the many formulations and techniques for achieving a calmer, more focused life. She might talk about the "five hindrances," examining each of the tendencies that prevent us from full absorption in the present and receptivity to the "enlightened" moment always available to us. She might delineate the "four foundations of mindfulness," beginning with mindfulness of the body. Or she might, over the course of a week-long retreat, lead us through the elements of the Eightfold Noble Path, the Buddha's prescription for attaining liberation.

But one of the most potent and engaging teaching methods Ruth used was her stories. Often not in the formal Dharma talk but spontaneously during the day, she would begin to recount an incident from her life. Some of the power of these stories came from her willingness to share her confusion and weakness as well as her strength, revealing her own human fallibility. Sometimes on those long days in the meditation hall, Ruth would begin a story. It would appear to wander and traverse many detours, but it always arrived at a moment that stuck in the mind, like an arrow pointing at something one had missed before or had never considered.

On one particular morning, after three hours of sitting and walking meditation, someone had asked Ruth about difficulties with the breathing practice.

"At some point you may find yourself not being able to breathe out," Ruth answered. "When the breath stops, some of the toxins stay in your body, and that builds up a great tension. Then you find congestion here, tremendous pain, and frustration arises in the mind. That is a very natural development in our breathing practice."

She cocked her head to the side, pondering. Morning light touched her strong-boned face.

"But if we stay attentive, with an open mind, without resenting or wishing—stay in attention with this kind of mind, which is very pure— then we are able to permit the breath to come to a very soft rhythm."

She leaned forward to peer challengingly at us.

"If our mind is open and free of resenting or wishing, we can allow the breath to come to its own naturalness, hmm? But somehow we can't just *do* that! The problem is that our mind runs along on its own way. We have very little control over it. Who notices this?"

A number of the meditators nodded.

She spoke of how the body's discomfort triggered the mind, frustration arose, and we then began to be emotional about that. Finally we doubted whether we would ever breathe again and whether we could do this practice, whether Buddhism was really "our thing" or if we should just give up and go to the beach: a whole drama ensued as we sat there trying to look serene.

People laughed in recognition.

"So I urge you to keep cool, not to indulge in those emotional reactions, simply watch what's going on, and do not doubt this practice."

Ruth sat back, adjusting the chain that held her eyeglasses hanging on her chest. "You may wonder whether, after all these years, I doubt this practice. I tell you I have tested it. There was a time in my life when I experienced extreme states of terror and pain because of difficulties with breathing."

A deeper silence fell among us as she continued.

"My difficulties had arisen from wrong practice," she said, leaning forward slightly, her face severe. "I had been too eager-beaver, I was concentrating too harshly, pushing it too hard in a determined way. So then there came a very great rebound to that. Over a period of a year was what I call the dark age of my practice. My mind suffered tremendously; it almost split off and was unmanageable for me. Unmanageable. I could not concentrate in any way. Today I know why I had to experience that. It brought me into a great space of humbleness and respect for myself, and love.

"But then all I knew was that I had no power over the mind. It just roamed around and created pictures and fear. Even the imagination suffered and was injured. All good faculties for sustaining mindfulness on breathing had gone off and been disassociated from me. Some of you are psychologists or social workers—you have probably met people in this condition, hmm?"

She looked out among us, nodding as someone indicated agreement. Then she clasped her hands before her and continued, "But I did not suffer doubt, because I could remember that this practice is good, and also I realized that my problem had come not because of any lack in the *practice,* but through my own wrongdoing. So I trusted. I began humbly returning to the practice, just being happy with a crumb, with the littlest thing I could achieve. Picking up the broom and understanding, 'I have the broom in my hand.' Or bending down and really telling myself several times, 'I am bending down.' I would tell myself, 'I have a nose.' I would touch it, rub it. I would put it into water. And realize, 'This nose permits the air to come through.'"

She paused, her body drawn up into alertness. I felt her extreme interest in that condition she had experienced, and an urgency that we should understand her.

"Because I was in training and I had good concentrative power and good practice, experiencing such a dilemma was not so dangerous. I didn't lose faith, and I didn't lose trust and confidence. So I could go to the lowest type of practice, the most modest one, to begin there, and I could gradually come back. That gave me wonderful ways of exploration that I can share with you now when I am teaching.

"But while it was going on, I couldn't even drive the car. I didn't have that kind of concentration. It was *serious*, my dear friends. The energies were in that much disharmony."

She looked around at the thirty or so of us.

"Through sharing this with you, maybe I can transmit the enormous importance of this practice, and the enormous sensitivity of this practice. The danger, too."

She explained that if we force the breath, pushing it out, "the outbreath can take the mind with it," leaving us disassociated. She reminded us that the Buddha did not tell us to strive to attain something in breathing but merely directed us to observe the breath just as it is. "This he did because he understood the healing power of the pure, unattached mind," she said, "this correcting power that demands nothing, and thus allows what you observe to come into its natural order again."

She adjusted herself on her seat and leaned back a little, her face relaxing. "So if you feel difficulties, pain, and congestion, don't be too much concerned. Be only concerned that your mind is pure, not reacting. Anything else will with time…it might take you twenty years…" and she laughed, "…will with time come into order. Now to *reduce* those twenty years a little…" this time it was the students who laughed "…I come in and invite you, with a quiet nondetermined mind or nonemotional mind, to just observe what you are doing. Watch how you breathe. Can you discover something in it? It is all for one reason, to train the mind to stay here, to invite it, hmm? To overcome some of the difficulties and give us more trust, to give us more confidence."

She paused, glancing out the glass doors at the side of the room, to the desert, where the chaparral dipped and tossed in the wind. The dirt gleamed yellowish in the hot sun and the apron of concrete glared whitely. As if they had been summoned by her attention, two black dogs arrived scrabbling and panting outside the screen to chase each other in a circle, and were gone again. Ruth smoothed the pleats in her skirt and rested her hands on her knees.

"So that was one of my difficulties. I tell you it was terror at times. I hear that often from you. You experience fear coming up because you feel you are now totally without breath." She chuckled. "Those who are more positive, they will say, 'Ah, I have no breath now, I am just about to get enlightened!' You see, that's also nonsense. That's just a sign of extreme absentmindedness. You don't even know where your mind is, but now to justify this you will say, 'I feel nothing; I am really pure: where is that enlightenment? I'm just ready for it!'" Ruth put back her head and gave herself up to the laughter beginning in the room.

Then gradually we became still again. She waited, looking into the faces before her, and finally spoke with great seriousness "I was in terror when I could not notice the breath. I really felt I'd died. So I would go to the trees in the garden and I would look at the leaves, just holding onto the thought, 'There is life and I am life too, and so if I can stay close to that thought and that expression of life I can survive a little longer.' But the fear came right back, and it was unbearable. In the night I consulted a high Zen master with whom I had been practicing in Los Angeles. When I asked him to come over to save me from dying, he gave me the message through the telephone that he cannot come because he is leading a retreat, and he tells me to die quietly. That was the message."

There was a rustle of shock in the room.

"I didn't quite get the message though. I asked for another master. I was at that time very much helping two Zen centers in Los Angeles get established, and I used their space for my practice. So that night at two o'clock, I called for the other Zen master, and he came. I was so distraught. Just looking at him gave me some connectedness. I described my state and he knew what was happening. He gave no help. He said, 'Let go. Don't try. Die.' And he left."

Ruth was sitting very still now, her hands cupped on her knees, her face lifted slightly. I felt a change in my breath, a sort of psychic drop, to a place somewhere between distress and awe.

"When he left it was then dawn. Two friends were there with me. I asked them to prepare for my dying." This time when she laughed, the students did not. Glancing around, I saw troubled, attentive faces. "And I let myself now really go into that experience...not holding on anymore, softening into that, falling into what is given at this moment. And I suddenly could notice. I observed my friends preparing, bringing beautiful lilies from the garden, pink lilies—amaryllis I think they are called. They brought candles in too. It was in my bedroom. And I just watched them and really followed the message both masters gave me, to let go. But I could kind of now understand that it was happening, and I asked my friends to read for me the *Bhagavad Gita* and part of the *Dhammapada* that is the wisdom teaching of the Buddha, and just listened to it, and I connected! Through listening to the words, I understood. I totally gave up any striving against, any want to be aware of the breath, any desire. I was determined to notice my dying, and what I noticed was my coming back to breathing. The body became very relaxed. I felt a total acceptance of the moment. And no fear was there."

I sensed the relief of the others in the room, as welcome as mine, at this outcome. And once again through this story the ancient dictum was repeated: in this moment be fully present to your own experience. How easy that sounds and yet how difficult, often terrifying, it is to do.

"From there on I was more available to myself," Ruth continued, "to work and re-establish mindfulness on breathing. It took about two years until I came back to the point where I had started. I called it my 'knitting time.' I knitted myself back together. When friends came to visit, I just said, 'I need now to retreat for my knitting time.' So you see, if we handle ourselves well, we can open up to our deeper self and allow those qualities to come and support us which make available this 'cool' of which I spoke."

Ruth finished slowly, bringing home the message.

"You allow the mind to come in with its desires, with all its conditioning, its compulsion to think, to strive, to resent, to want, and so on. And then you are really an explorer. You are noticing all this coming in and not forbidding it, not pushing it away but permitting it to live in the light of your attention. Remember this vipassana mind, this witnessing, attending mind, is already part of your beautiful self. So if you can hold onto that in a modest way you can sustain that cool. You can provide again and again a beautiful condition for your practice."

She lifted her head, looking to the back of the room where I sat, and inquired briskly, "Does that make sense to you, Sandy?"

I thought for a moment. "Yes, it does," I said.

"Good." Ruth gave a decisive nod. "I hope it makes sense to all of us."

9

On the Gurney

*The kind of discoveries that are made through Buddhist practice
have nothing to do with believing in anything. They have
much more to do with having the courage to die,
the courage to die continually.*

Pema Chodron

LIKE A MIST curtaining from the surface of a black deep pond, I rise up
into voices, slabs of hard sound, scrapes of metal, thuds and clinks. I realize that I lie on my side. Just across from me, on a wheeled table like
mine, in this huge brightness that allows us no modest hiding of blem-
ish or sag, looking back at me is a man as dark as the pond from which
I have risen. But his skin, unlike that deadness, gathers the light, gleaming with highlights of warm mahogany. He is trying to pull himself to a
sitting position, his elbows jabbing air and the hospital gown falling back
to expose his wrinkled thigh. No one comes to help us, we're utterly
alone with each other here in the bowels of Highland Hospital, the long
crowded corridor and warren of rooms that is Emergency.

Then we are joined by an intern clutching a clipboard. She has a lovely
Asian face, like Kwan Yin.

"What symptoms are you having?" she asks me.

I can't quite manage a response. A few weeks after my trip to Point
Reyes, one day I had begun to vomit and then could not stop: didn't I
already tell two groups of interns about this?

I lie back, imagining this white-coated young woman in the elaborate
headdress and flowing robe that Kwan Yin wears, her dress blown by the
sea wind. Kwan Yin of the South Seas, savior of fishermen—help me
through this storm. In ancient times, in each of the bays and inlets of

Southern China, there resided a local goddess. She would be called upon in the midst of rain and lightning and violent seas to rescue fishermen from danger. When Buddhism came to China, these salvific female figures were reborn as Kwan Yin.

My week of not eating and regular retching did feel like a perilous journey. Racked by my body's revulsion, I had found my capacity to meditate fading away. I arrived in a condition beyond choice and discernment. If I was still an actor in my own drama—that pale, ethereal production, it went something like this: imagine looking at a stage, dim and shrouded, with willow trees, a distant moon, and a fountain amid dark shrubs, a spooky nineteenth-century stage set, fit for the appearance of ghosts. Then, enter a shadowy figure who announces in a thready voice, "I will try to eat again." Trying to eat was the only willed action I had participated in for the last several days; the rest—the vomiting, the falling asleep and waking up—all happened by itself.

Still, I am able to see this intern, whose mouth is pursing with impatience, as a graceful embodiment of the quality of compassion. She could be an actress in that drama, hovering there among the willow branches as Kwan Yin does in representations on Putuo Shan, looking down at the human being who calls upon her.

"What seems to be wrong with you?" the intern repeats, and I am brought abruptly back to the gurney on which I lie.

Somehow speechless, I look around for help. Glancing down to the foot of the gurney I'm relieved to see Crystal, but she appears so pale and tired that she frightens me.

"She's been vomiting for seven days," Crystal informs the intern. I have a momentary image of the days passed at home, lying weakly in bed, watching Crystal take the pan to empty, and bring it back; accepting the simple food she would bring me later, as we both hoped I could keep it down. No wonder she looks so exhausted, I thought, for she had also accepted a commission to compose another choral work, due in a few months, and was juggling my care with that pressured creative labor. Now, seeing her standing there, her face strained in the brutal neon glare, I am filled with gratitude, and wish I could make things easier for her.

But my stomach interrupts. I feel it lift, my esophagus clench, tighten, and then surrender. Next to me on the gurney, I see, is a shallow metal pan. I lift my head and let the foamy liquid erupt out of my throat and splash into the pan.

"Cancer," says Crystal to the intern, "Chemotherapy."

My white-coated Kwan Yin and her cohorts write on their clipboards, their smooth foreheads earnest.

When they have left, I wonder if I am smiling at Crystal. I would like to express my thanks that she is here. It's a softness in my chest, but I don't know if my face smiles.

After the difficult day at Point Reyes Crystal was kind to me, and the next morning left a card on my pillow that read:

> *I'm sorry you're feeling so poorly.*
> *I'm sorry I didn't wait till you were feeling better to "come unglued."*
> *Guess the seams were holding everything in—until all this upset, pressure and all—then it broke.*
> > *I still love you very much, Crystal.*

So the weeks went, with Crystal gentle with me one day and angry at me the next. When she came into the bedroom each night from her hours of composing, she would be too wound up to sleep, and would turn on the television and spread her business papers across the bed.

During this last week of vomiting and weakness Crystal had cared for me tenderly, worrying about me as I grew weaker. Finally she began to fear that I was dying, and called the Wandering Menstruals to help her decide what to do.

Now, looking up at her white, distracted face, I ask, "When did we get here?"

"The Menstruals brought you over at about three o'clock. It's eleven now."

"Have you been here all this time?" My voice comes lazily, words issuing without force, drifting in the air.

"Only for a little while. When I came Sandy Butler was here."

Beyond the curtain comes a burst of noise. Voices, running feet: they're pushing someone past, yelling at each other, clamp this, pump that! Panic like a great bird flaps in the hall—I feel the wind of its wings on my cheeks.

Having sunk into the still, dark pool again, I come up to consciousness to see that the gurney across from me is occupied this time by an old woman. Kindness and care have carved shallow gullies on her face; she looks as if her back and limbs are electric with pain as she holds onto the hard workman's hands of a young man who resembles her. His dark head is tilted close to hers, his face, bigger and coarser than hers, contorted in equal distress. I feel tears pooling at the sight of them.

"What seems to be the problem?" asks an African-American young man in his stiff snowy coat.

Yes, what is it? I ask myself. What terrible disease wracks this woman? How has she come here to this place in such agony? And will she find help? Is there a shot or a pill or....

The intern leans closer to me and raises his eyebrows. Slowly I realize he is asking about me, about *my* "problem."

Each time I arrive out of my darkness into consciousness, I become more aware of the noises, the endless bustle, clangs, bumps, and tense raised voices outside my curtained cubicle.

Next to my gurney now stands Deborah. I am so glad to see her round, kind face, to feel her hand stroking my arm. Deborah tells me, because she is a nurse and knows these things, that the drug dripping into my hand through the IV has stopped the vomiting.

"And see this bag? They're puttin' fluids in you for your dehydration. I bet they'll take you upstairs to a hospital room pretty soon and you can rest."

Rolling her eyes toward some new uproar in the hall outside our curtain, Deborah grins. "I guess you been havin' *some* night, huh?"

I feel my lips pulling up into an answering grin. "I guess so."

Strange, but after this long night I feel completely at one with the great anthill of Highland Hospital, like a creature whose true environment is the lower depths. As I did at Point Reyes, where I breathed and opened to awareness of my interconnection with ocean, shore and sky, I have surrendered to my surroundings here in the ground-floor emergency room. The floors of the hospital rise above me—hundreds of people move and talk, bend and lift; hands touch roughly or with a practiced tenderness—as I lie here in the fundament, like the tumor that inhabited my colon, growing silent and unnoticed in the dark. I can't imagine being anywhere but here, absorbed into this giant body.

But I do wonder about the passage of time, which is impossible to gauge in this fluorescent eternity.

"Deborah, how late is it?"

She lifts her hand from my arm to look at her big-faced nurse's watch. "It's 3:30 in the morning."

I stare in astonishment at her as I calculate. I have been on this hard gurney for twelve hours. The thought plunges me into a puddle of weakness. And yet my head, arms, and chest buzz, perhaps from the drug they've been giving me or the palpable tension around me, or maybe from not having had any nourishment for seven days except this drip of liquid into the vein on the back of my hand. I know I am in an unusual condition, unhinged by the anguish I have seen here, the perpetual haste and crisis heard through that yellow curtain.

I try to focus on my breath, to experience the flow of warm air over my upper lip as I inhale, the touch of breath on my nostrils—to experience life where it is actually taking place. But abruptly, a doctor appears. As though springing up from the floor, he materializes next to me. He is erect, brisk, blond with little mouse-tufts of gray at his temples. Is this a senior doctor, or yet another in the parade of interns who have looked in on me during the night?

He consults the clipboard lifted from my gurney.

"Well, Ms. Boo-cher, looks like you're stabilized. I'll get the nurse to send you upstairs and we'll keep you until tomorrow to make sure you're done with that vomiting."

And he's gone.

Deborah pats my arm.

Zing of the curtain whipping open, and a nurse enters. Her thighs stretch the legs of her white pantsuit; she looks dead-tired but determined.

"They'll be sending someone down for you soon. Till then, I'm putting you in the hallway."

The hallway! Deborah looks as stricken as I feel.

"Oh no, please," I beg. "Don't put me there."

"It won't be long," the nurse answers. She leans to release the brake on the gurney, and I find myself gliding out of my curtained haven, a sacrificial victim in a wicked sorcerer's canoe, pushed from shore into a crocodile-infested stream. For the second time tonight I am afraid; fluttering wings beat inside my chest, brushing my ribs.

Gurneys line the walls of this bright loud corridor. Nurses and interns rush through a collision course of crutches, wheelchairs, and IV stands. Patients lie swollen, bloodied, with great angry bruises, wearing patches of gauze hastily stuck over the holes in their skins; rent, opened, struck down by a cramping heart, a drug-induced mental full-stop. Some twist and moan. Policemen lounge at the entrance, radiating authority.

The nurse parks my gurney against the wall, and I am becalmed in this place I was so afraid of entering. The wings in my chest flutter to a halt, leaving an expectant silence in their wake. Deborah finds a chair and sits at the head of my gurney with her arm up next to my pillow; and I realize she is familiar and comfortable with this hospital world. Perhaps she can be my guide, like a bodhisattva in the hell realm, ready to offer the remedy of awakening to the agonized inhabitants. Together we look out over this wreckage of broken, beaten people.

The gurney just in front of me is occupied by a rawboned blond woman. She looks to be about forty, a jeans-clad, hard-luck looking woman with a puffy purpled face and stiff bleached hair. She's sitting up, but her wrists and ankles are held tight to the metal bars by thick leather straps.

"God damn you, let me up! I've pee'd my pants! I'm sittin' here in my own piss." Her voice clangs, thick and metallic.

"Nurse!" she shouts to someone pushing past her, "Nurse, you got to let me up! Unfasten me!" She jerks her arms against the straps.

"On her way to the psycho ward," mutters the nurse as he passes. "Tried to kill somebody and then herself."

I feel a quaking inside. I can't stand this—I can't stand anymore! All night I've been filled and filled with it, and now I have room for no more.

"Help!" she shouts. "Let me up off here. Nurse! Nurse!"

Her frenzy enters me and pushes against the last fragile threads of my control. It hurts more than I can believe for a long, long few minutes.

And then something trembles, rips, and falls away. And I feel myself pass through. Suddenly I am in a realm where all has become wide and still. I have lost what solidity I had, and instead become a shower of musical notes tinkling like glass in the silence. Maybe this is the realm that Kwan Yin inhabits, beyond my usual perceptions and expectations, beyond boundaries—the truth explored in the Heart Sutra, that "form does not differ from emptiness; emptiness does not differ from form."

This goes beyond my penetration into the flow of phenomena, which I have entered in meditation, where I have been aware of my body as atoms gyrating, as waves of energy endlessly transmuting. No, this is something else, as if all of me has been lifted out into a vast space that is both inside me and outside containing me. A space that encompasses every person, object, sound and smell, holding all in exquisite pleasurable suspension.

I look questioningly into Deborah's brown eyes; she smiles, and I wonder if she is here with me in this same condition.

Then I sink back, aware that there is nothing I could want that could match this fullness. A plethora of joys vibrates in the huge space that I inhabit and have become.

I look around me, seeing the tired tense faces of the nurses and the young interns, seeing a man lying deathly still with a huge white bandage on his head, a young man in a wheelchair huddled over his bloody leg, a woman clutching a sobbing child. Their distress enters this spaciousness and hovers, held in a radiance of infinite tenderness.

The woman on the gurney before me continues to rant. "You fuckers, you get me off this thing and let me go to the bathroom! Nurse! Nurse! I tell you I pee'd my pants here, I'm sittin' in a goddamned puddle, damn you, I'm gonna flood this whole damned hallway!"

The woman does not know that Deborah and I are laughing. Together, helpless before this onslaught, we have slipped beyond suffering and compassion and bodies and instruments, beyond noise, blood, and pain. Giggling, we acknowledge the limitless absurdity of all of it, including ourselves—I with the big scar in my belly and my veins full of chemicals, Deborah plunged with me into this cauldron among the interns punchy with fatigue, the deliberate nurses and harried clerks, the restless policemen itching to leave—all of us shimmering in this heightened light, gone so far beyond our minds and bodies into the immense, loving welcome of the universe.

PART THREE

10

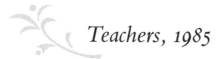

Teachers, 1985

Our life's work is to use what we have been given to wake up.
Pema Chodron

I<small>T WAS AT</small> D<small>HAMMA</small> D<small>ENA</small> that I first heard about *dukkha*, the Buddha's First Noble Truth. Learning that new word, rolling it on my tongue, I did not want to admit its gritty truth. But over time, sitting in the small crowded meditation hall that was all we had then, I experienced the restlessness, anger, and stubborn resistance that ruled my life, the insistence that things be other than they were, and I knew this to be *dukkha*. Ruth taught us to redirect the urge to escape our suffering; she guided us into the sensations of each successive moment, trained us to bring our attention there and to simply watch our busy thoughts and unruly emotions before returning again into attention to our sensory experience.

Still, for three years I had resisted Ruth, fighting her in order to preserve the familiar, desire-ridden, out-of-control self that caused me so much suffering. It was a life and death struggle, for Ruth threatened me with the death—at any moment—of my concepts and opinions, my self-construction. I exerted all my power against her and made myself miserable to protect my little self-referential identity. I went to Ruth because I could no longer bear to live in such a limited way, and yet I could not open to her. This struggle went on like a war raging in me, stifling me, continually thwarting my efforts to concentrate, meditate, and be simply present. During those years I saw how much of my suffering was self-created; I experienced the tremendous power of my conditioned responses.

Perhaps I could have continued my internal war for decades, if I had not found myself utterly without money as a retreat-session drew near. I telephoned Dhamma Dena and explained my predicament. Was there a way, I asked, that I could attend the retreat for free? Half an hour later, someone called back to convey Ruth's message that I was welcome to work for my room and board.

So I spent hours each day at Dhamma Dena painting and cleaning and building. And I began to experience myself joined with my surroundings. I became part of the physical reality of structures, carpets, and windows; I entered the energy of the place, promoting its continued existence and creating order. And I began to be wholly committed to each task; that embattled self was forgotten, and I knew only the action of hand holding rag wiping wall.

One particular labor tried my endurance. I dug a hole for a latrine, bending over the shovel and lifting the clods of heavy dirt within sight of the meditation hall, where the other retreatants sat peacefully in meditation. A cold wind battered me; the wooden handle of the shovel wore against the skin of my hands, raising blisters; and my back began to ache. In the performance of this task, at last the carapace of my resistance broke apart. After hours of shoveling, I entered the hall and lowered my body onto my cushion with immense relief. To sit still, to meditate, seemed a great privilege and gift in itself. Looking to Ruth at the front of the room, I saw her anew: not as my tormentor, but as one who offered a precious opportunity. I saw that she was always gently pointing to the authenticity of this moment, suggesting a new way for me to be with my experience. I surrendered utterly to her teaching, opening to receive her directions—no longer shutting my heart and mind to them but letting them enter me—and I was profoundly touched. I *saw* Ruth, all her skill, insight and love for us that she gave, without holding back anything, in order to awaken in us the capacity to open to our own freedom. In those few days, all the teachings of the previous three years that I had so vigorously rejected jelled in me. I felt myself enter a deep and enduring life-force, expansive and sure, and full of a quiet joy.

This is not to say that I was totally transformed. Even now sometimes, my resistance will pop up to impede me. Resistance is a habit, and it is hard instead to patiently attend to what is going on. But there was a qualitative change during that retreat that left me much more receptive to and able to make use of Ruth's teachings.

On one spring retreat, after the noon meal I left the little cluster of buildings that was Dhamma Dena to hike out toward the mountains. As I walked among the scattered bushes, I startled small lizards who were the same color as the crumbly tan earth. There were no sounds out here but the crunch of my footsteps under the rush of the wind. But if I stood still, I could also hear the buzz of flies, and saw a fat bee visiting a blossom of a creosote bush.

Ruth's story about the time when she had lost contact with herself and had had to knit herself back together, her willingness to open herself to us in so vulnerable a way, had affected me strongly. I was pondering her message of surrender to life, and even to death, when a jackrabbit leapt from the shade of a sage bush ahead of me and went hopping away, its ears high. Acutely now I was aware of my cohabitation with the animals of the desert, with the very dirt and plants. I considered that there was no question of surrender in a lizard's life; it was neither blessed nor burdened with many choices, cursed nor graced with the ability to resist what was given.

Crossing the indentation of a rarely used road, I came upon a concrete square that had once been the floor of a house. A skeletal couch sat there now, its rusted wire hung with two mats of stuffing, gray and fluffy, like patches of hair on an old man's chest. Everything had been stripped away by the mice, kangaroo rats, and birds. Broken bottles and odd bits of wood were strewn across the concrete, which shone so brightly in the sun that I had to squint. On the ground around the foundation lay shingles and tarpaper, most of it to the east of the platform, as though the wind had pushed the walls and roof over and scattered them across the ground.

Now I realized that I was hearing the mutter of a pickup truck, which had arrived behind me and sat idling on the road. As I turned to look, the woman in the cab waved me over.

Walking across the desert toward her, I saw her round tanned face peer out at me from under the floppy brim of a straw hat as I came close.

"Hullo! You that lady from the city interested in this place?"

Having established that I was only a visitor, not a prospective buyer, the woman told me, "I just been down to Joshua Tree to the parade for Turtle Days. I live right over there by the hills."

Her freckled hands rested on the steering wheel. She looked full into my face with friendly eyes.

"Who you visitin'? Ruth who? Does she help out over at the fire house occasionally? We had a real nice hamburger roast over there a while back. D'you think I'd of met her there?"

I said a few things about Ruth, being careful, for I knew that she did not want to appear too exotic to the people of Copper Mountain Mesa.

When the woman's pickup had shrunk into the distance, I went on with my walk. Ruth had told me that many of the residents of this mesa were retired people, some who had built their houses back when all you had to do was come out here, stake a claim, and build a cabin at least twelve by eight feet—and the land on which it stood would be yours. Ruth came much later, during a period when she and her husband Henry were separated. In the preceding years, she and Henry had gone camping together in the mountains. Ruth did not feel safe camping alone, so she had bought the little main house with outbuildings as a place in which to escape the city. The meditation hall, Dukkha House, and several other smaller houses farther away had been acquired later.

As I approached the mountains, I saw Joshua trees tilted like perform-ing mimes, fixed in odd postures against the sky. They stood so much taller than the surrounding chaparral, and were each so uniquely formed, shaggy on their trunks and spiky on top, that visiting each tree was like meeting some hoary old prospector or a scarred, weathered desert rat with stories to tell.

The foothills of the mountains, when I got closer, were transformed into rounded-off piles of huge brown rocks, with a few tiny houses perched here and there among them. Some of these were cabins for hunters, I knew.

Out to the east was a spread, with small house and gleaming silver tank truck pulled up under the tree next to a trailer. On this desert, you dug down about three feet and hit a layer of rock so thick that sinking a well was extremely expensive. Everyone bought water and had it trucked out from town, storing it in tanks that stood near the houses of the peo-ple who lived here year 'round. The hunters and vacation people got along on bottled water.

I sat to rest under a Joshua tree, looking back in the direction of Dhamma Dena, which had disappeared into the flat earth. Far beyond, the mountains stood softly outlined within a light blue haze.

The sun was hot on my shoulders and knees, but the wind was cool.

This wind could be so abrasive at times, but now, without it, the sun and heat out here would have been unbearable. I was thinking still of Ruth's story, how she had said that the experience of that anguished period had humbled her, teaching her to start again with the most elementary steps to attain concentration.

There was usually at least one person at each retreat who was in obvious psychological trouble. A relative or friend would have heard that what we were doing at Dhamma Dena might be helpful, and they would bring the person there, get them registered, and disappear. Often the person was incapable of sitting still for meditation, so Ruth would find a task that would engage a wandering mind. One young man had looked terrified, his eyes glancing everywhere, his motions quick and jerky. Ruth showed him how to rake the sandy dirt of the yard in long curves, as if a lazy hand were dragging its fingers in the dirt. When I came through the yard I would see him there, raking with increasing care, and as the week progressed his fear gradually lessened. He seemed to find some peace in this simple activity, some reliable focus, and even pleasure. Now I understand that Ruth was able to work with people in mental distress because of her own experience.

The same applied to her work with the rest of us, in our varying degrees of mental distress. Her teaching, so grounded in what she knew, had great stability and power. She was especially gifted in her explorations of the body, for she seemed preternaturally sensitive to physical sensations, able to penetrate with great thoroughness and subtlety into the living reality of her own human experience. Perhaps it was this constant exploration that evoked the compassion and insight we experienced from her, and which allowed her to approach each living being with equal respect.

I leaned back against the scratchy trunk of the Joshua tree, adjusting my buttocks on the piled rocks at its base, and thought about what I received from Ruth. First, the support of knowing I could always begin again, return to the simplest practice—as she had done with the broom: "This is a broom, and I am sweeping"—to reconnect with the living moment-to-moment process of my life. Over the years that I had come here to sit with her, I had learned that each contact in my life was an opportunity to practice, which implied that each being, human or otherwise, whom I encountered, was my teacher. Ruth Denison spoke with great veneration of her Buddhist teacher, the Burmese master U Ba Khin, and an oil painting of him in brown monk's robes hung on the wall of the meditation hall. But each of her stories conveyed her gratitude for the many teachers she encountered in daily life.

Unlike some other forms of Buddhism, in which devotion to the teacher is a primary part of the practice, in Theravada Buddhism the teacher is seen simply as a "spiritual friend." The Buddha himself became angry when a follower displayed too much attachment to his person: he instructed that it was the teachings that mattered, not the human being who delivered them. In Buddhist art, the Buddha at first was not depicted, or was represented by an empty seat, for it was his absence, not presence, that was significant: he had become fully realized so that when his body died he was truly gone, never to be reborn into human or other form.

Still, since we are human beings with ordinary needs, we honor our teachers, project our desires onto them, resist, surrender to, and struggle with them. For some people I know, it has made sense to move from one spiritual teacher to another, seeking out that yet-more-illumined guide who can take them to the next step in their practice. For me, although I had sat with numerous teachers, it felt right to stay loyal to one teacher, for I understood that a teacher is a mirror, reflecting one back to oneself. Staying with the same mirror over time had allowed me to see patterns in myself and how they changed. Ruth remained herself, offering teachings in the ways she had developed; I came to her each time experiencing her and myself differently, learning new things and going deeper.

For example, my response to Uliloo when he came waddling and coughing into the meditation hall this morning: I had lost my focus and tensed up, because of the concept I held that a dog does not belong in a meditation hall. I had seen the tendency in myself to want things to be orderly and predictable, and to render judgment when the unexpected arrives. Ridiculous, particularly since I knew the story of how Uliloo became a teacher to Ruth.

Thirteen years before, Ruth had been suffering back trouble that required a lengthy operation and confinement in a full-body cast. The drugs and anesthesia had affected her so drastically that she once again lost her connection to her own breathing. She was frightened, especially when she was brought home and left essentially alone. (Henry at that time was, as she put it, "flying around the world somewhere wanting to find his happiness.") A friend did come to feed and care for her, but was too frightened of her condition to stay with her for long periods.

In Los Angeles at that time a major earthquake occurred. Ruth lay in bed one morning alone in the house, and suddenly everything started to move. From the mantel of the fireplace objects began to fall onto her bed. Around her everything shook, and the ceiling rippled in waves above her. Since she didn't know anything about earthquakes, in the beginning she thought it was her own mind playing tricks on her. In the afternoon an acquaintance came to visit, saying that because their house had been destroyed by the earthquake, they wanted to give away their litter of dachshund puppies—and would she take one? In her loneliness, Ruth said yes.

The frightened puppy needed company and whined alone in the corner. Finally Ruth coaxed him to her bed. She picked him up and placed him upon her chest, just under her chin—he was as small as a rat—and talked babytalk to him, saying how afraid he must be to be away from his mama, and how afraid she was too. It did her good. Even in her distress, she remembered the principle of always being aware of what you did. All she could be aware of at this point was that this little creature was on her chest. She said it to herself, fully realized it, noticing, I am alive, I'm here. Then she noticed him falling asleep, breathing evenly. "He thought he was on his mother's belly," Ruth explained, and the warmth of another body lulled him. Ruth paid attention to the rhythm of his breathing as he slept, following it in and out. Somehow she allowed her chest to rise and fall with his. So as they did this breathing practice together, she was able to reestablish her sense of being alive. In this she had seen the little dog as her teacher, and had developed a grateful affection for him.

Scrambling up from my seat under the Joshua tree, I brushed off my pants and started back. I walked slowly across the dry earth, hearing it crunch under my shoes, observing the holes made by the rabbits and desert tortoises at the bases of the creosote bushes. Uliloo himself was not much bigger than the jackrabbits.

At the same time as his arrival, she told us, she had received a notice that her teacher in Burma, U Ba Khin, had died. Ruth scoffed at the coincidence: "You can put a lot of thoughts into it and emotions, and so on...it was just what it was...people die at the time you get a little dog."

But still, she sometimes called the dog U Ba Khin, and always treated him with special care.

Now the buildings of Dhamma Dena appeared over a rise, and I saw Ruth, a small figure, her skirt unfurling in the wind, absorbed in earnest conversation with the cook outside the kitchen door.

I hurried to arrive at the meditation hall and take my seat on a cushion before Ruth arrived. And I thought about gratitude, her gratitude to Uliloo, to U Ba Khin, to so many others—how her acknowledgment of what had been given to her permeated her whole life.

11

"We're Family in Here"

*…we encourage ourselves to develop an open heart and an
open mind, to heaven, to hell, to everything.*
Pema Chodron

JULIA CHILD stands a little to the side of the butcher block, her face radiating indulgent interest, as a young man chops celery and talks about how to begin making a shitake mushroom soup. "And you've already fried a bit of bacon," Julia prompts.

"Yes, and now the carrots and the potatoes," he says, pushing aside the celery.

I glance sideways at my roommate. Sonya sits in her cranked up bed, erect as a queen, gazing with ardent eyes at the goings-on in Julia's Kitchen. Cooking shows are Sonya's favorite, and, ever courteous, she is relieved that I profess to like them too. We watch in companionable silence: Sonya never comments on anything she sees. In my first few days here my attempts to discover her opinion elicited only a gracious, dreamy smile, so I gave up.

The young man has removed the stems from the mushrooms and tossed them into the frying pan with the other vegetables. Bacon grease sizzles delectably as Julia, looming next to the man, makes good-natured comments on his work.

I think about the soup that will result. I think about eating. With the tube through my nose and down my throat, I am not allowed to eat or drink. I know Sonya is unaware of the difficulty of watching a cooking show when one cannot eat, and I forgive her. She is a woman beset with cravings, so busy with them that quite a few things escape her notice.

"Now for the stock," Julia encourages, and the young man ladles in some liquid from a plastic container.

After the last harrowing hospitalization, I was moderately comfortable for a few days. Then extreme stomach pain began, and the surgeons suspected a problem at the place where they had stitched my bowel back together. I could not eliminate, and the pain became unbearable. Here in the hospital room, nurses arrive periodically to give me enemas—three so far today. (Does this rubber bag full of soapy water truly reflect the sophistication of modern medicine?) Then the surgeons gather around my bed to discuss my case. They speak of "adhesions," or a "kink in your bowel." One of them peered at me through spectacles and said, "We hope to unkink it." Five days of this—long enough for me to get to know Sonya.

"Salt and pepper," announces the young man as he shakes them on with a flourish.

"And to finish," says Julia, "a pinch of parsley and a dab of margarine."

The camera moves in close to the bowl of steaming soup. It looks delicious.

"Hey, pretty good," I comment, turning to Sonya.

She gazes blissfully back at me.

Sonya is a delicately built young woman with sleepy eyes, and Q-tip-thin brown legs under her hospital gown. One arm is slender, the other swollen to sausage girth and stuffed into an elastic sleeve. "It's from my mastectomy," she told me, wincing as she moved her monster arm, trying to find a comfortable way to position it in the sling the nurse had rigged for her. She seems so young, and told me that a friend had brought her six-year-old son to visit her yesterday. She had gone down to the lobby to see him. "I got to hold my baby and kiss him." Her face opened in joy.

Sonya sleeps at odd times, nodding off in the midst of an exchange with me. We don't have conversations exactly: she tells me about herself. Like this morning. Sonya slept through her breakfast. Tortured by the smell, I coveted her toast and eggs while she lay with her head lolling and mouth open.

When she finally awoke, Sonya was inexplicably annoyed at the breakfast. She stared disgustedly down at the contents of the plates. "I can't eat this!" she complained. "This is the worst breakfast I've ever seen!" Frowning indignantly, she pushed the buzzer for the nurse.

As we waited, she told me that she missed her alcohol. Holding my eyes with a level gaze, she said, "I drink every day at home." She let that sink in and then asked, "You know Cisco?"

I admitted my ignorance.

"It's wine, that's what I drink." She spoke wistfully, as though about a faraway lover. "I have me a bottle of Cisco in the morning, one in the afternoon, and two at night."

I try to imagine how that looks: Sonya at the kitchen table, drinking; in front of the TV set, drinking; on the front stoop. I wonder how that fits with mothering her little boy.

"I ain't violent or anything," she assures me. "But if I don't get my alcohol I get irritable."

I have seen how anxious she can get, thrashing in the bed, loudly demanding painkillers and sleeping pills. "Nurse, I need some Valium! Nurse, bring me Demerol!" Then she lowers her head, cradling her swollen arm and muttering many motherfuckers and goddamns and shits under her breath.

Now I understand this agitation as the addiction withdrawal symptom it is. Sonya's suffering is palpable, and I wait with her for the nurse to come and relieve her with a shot or a pill.

Medicated, she opens up with a sweetness that is totally engaging. She speaks to everyone, making friends, and she takes care of me. "We're family in here," she told me on the first day. "We have to watch out for each other." On her cigarette breaks, she tells me, she wanders the hospital wards, especially favoring the floor with the infants, where she looks in on each baby.

When the nurse comes in to give me another enema, pulling the curtain between us, Sonya disappears from sight. She never refers to my problems with my reluctant gut. Later, when I rush to the bathroom, dragging my IV stand with me, and shut the door, I am met with the reek of cigarette tobacco, sharp enough to pierce my chemo-damaged muffled sense of smell. Nausea rises in my throat.

Coming out to climb wearily into the bed, I say to Sonya, "You've been smoking in the john."

She glances drowsily at me, shrugs her good shoulder. "Yeah, sometimes I can't make it downstairs fast enough."

I am left to ponder desire—Sonya's and my own—the clinging and craving that cause us such suffering. In Buddhism we speak of the realm of *samsara,* the endless circling from suffering to desire to more suffering, which occasions more desire. The image representing *samsara* is a wheel, an ancient Indian symbol for the eternal round of conditioned existence alternating birth and death. The wheel is turned by the energy of our desire for ego satisfactions of every kind, our unceasing appetite, or *tanha* (thirst). The goal of the Buddha's teachings is to liberate us not from ordinary existence or the phenomenal world, but from the patterns of thought and behavior that enslave us. It is said that to fully realize *samsara* is to achieve *nirvana,* or enlightenment. The two realms are one, and the effort is to transform one's consciousness so as to break the chain of conditioned responses.

When we begin the practice of meditation, we become aware of the workings of *samsara.* I can observe it in myself, here in the bed. The tube in my nose hurts, and so I want it to be taken out; the more I resist its presence the more it hurts. The needle in the vein in my hand burns, and so I want it removed. I want the pain in my gut to disappear, and I want to eat and drink again. When my mind focuses on my discomfort, it manufactures desire, the fervent wish for things to be other than they are.

I realize this is not much different from my ordinary suffering within daily life—so many moments of wanting something other than what is happening.

So I close my eyes and bring my attention to the reality I am actually experiencing. I let myself feel the weight of my body in the bed, the pressure of the tube against my nostril and inside my throat, the pulling of the needle in my vein. As I pay attention to the sensations in my nose and hand, I begin to realize that they are fluctuating, vibrating, and I become more interested in the sensations than in my distress. The sensations—of pressure, of heat—continue, but I am no longer resisting them or defining them as discomfort or pain. Gradually, I experience them merely as sensations. Then I shift my focus to the breath, following it in and out, letting my mind move with it, all the way in through my nose and throat, then back out. After some minutes of this, I have arrived more strongly here where I am, and feel calmed.

I realize that Sonya is talking to me. I open my eyes to see her holding up the remote control.

"Let's cut it on and have us some nice TV. Want to?"

She smiles charmingly, and I suspect this is a gesture of apology for the cigarette smoke in the toilet.

"Sure."

We find ourselves observing Molly Katzen, author of the *Moosewood Cookbook*, concocting an Indian dinner.

Sonya is immediately engrossed, and I know there will be no more talking until Molly has chopped up lots of garlic and mixed it in the cooked yellow split peas to make dahl. We watch her add black pepper, crushed red pepper, mustard seed, turmeric, coriander, cumin seeds, and cinnamon.

Earlier I had asked Sonya if she liked to cook, only to receive a vague shrug. Did she like to eat exotic food? Again she shrugged, as if I were asking the wrong question. Perhaps what fascinates her, I speculate, is the care that is expressed here; perhaps she grew up watching her mother or her grandmother cook, providing for the family and Sonya herself, so that cooking shows coax her back into a warm, reassuring dependency.

I entertain these thoughts as Molly Katzen dribbles lemon juice over the dahl and salts it, and tells us it is best eaten with chapatis, thin pancake-like breads. As I watch and think, my sense of my body remains as a background. I feel strongly connected to the living process of my physical self.

Molly sets the dahl aside and begins the preparation for the rice pilaf; my mind wanders back to yesterday, when I saw Sonya's fierceness. It had been a hard night, with a lot of noise from a neighboring room, where a man sang and laughed wildly. The nurse told us he was a "5150," a psychiatric patient, with broken bones, who could not be moved to the psych ward until a doctor "signed him off." During the night Sonya had persuaded the nurse to give her a shot of Valium, and she became downright cheerful. But I was worried and irritable, for the machine that sucked brown acids from my stomach through the nose tube had stopped working. I imagined the acids burning into my stomach lining as I pushed the bell and complained to Sonya. Finally, when no help came, Sonya sprang from her bed and, head up, puffy arm cradled against her side, she announced, "I'm goin' down there and get you a nurse!" She sailed out of the room, gown flapping behind her narrow buttocks.

I lay back and found myself suddenly crying, the tears crawling hotly down my cheeks. When Sonya returned she stood at our doorway, alternately gazing reassuringly at me and peering imperiously down the hall in the direction of the nurse's station. In a few minutes a nurse arrived to adjust the machine and get it working again. When she had gone, drying my tears, I thanked Sonya, who didn't seem to hear me.

Now we watch Molly Katzen add almonds, walnuts, and raisins to the rice pilaf, and grate some lemon peel over the top, while Sonya smiles with satisfaction and deep interest. Mentally I thank her again, for being a teacher to me, fragile as she is, pulled about like a dandelion puff in the wind, and yet so generously loyal to life.

12

Weathering the Winter

*We have to stop gobbling this and pursuing that in our
shortsighted way, and simply relax into the cocoon, into
the darkness of the pain that is our life.*
Joko Beck

RELEASED FROM THE HOSPITAL AGAIN, I began the many months of
chemotherapy. Each Tuesday afternoon at the Hematology/Oncology
Clinic, I received an infusion of poison. There really is something ghoul-
ish about this whole chemotherapy routine. It smacks of a horror flick,
Bela Lugosi curling his finger in invitation, muttering "Come heeere," as
you sit down to allow the mysterious potion to enter and mingle with
your blood. After which, as in horror films, you will be transformed, and
not for the better. It's a dangerous maneuver: chemo and cancer wage war
inside your body, and the battle may kill you.

But the bearer of this infusion was far from the Bela Lugosi model. Bill
Shanks, the first person to give me the chemo, was a brown-skinned,
nattily dressed man with gray hair whose smile lit up the clinic. I soon
discovered that he was just my age, and hailed from Ohio like me. But it
was his hands that were most reassuring: broad, warm hands, whose
fingers moved deftly as he inserted the needle, with the skill learned in
years of this work and an innate gentleness that could not be learned.
Even so, I felt a sinking in my stomach as the clear liquid moved through
the needle from a vial into a vein on the back of my hand.

Each week a different friend accompanied me to sit on the plastic chairs
and wait, sometimes for three or four hours. The Oncology Clinic occupied the same set of rooms as the surgery and orthopedic clinics, so we
sat on that same row of chairs in the hallway, facing those same numbered

doors. Most everyone sitting there looked ill and unhappy: gray-skinned, weak, thin, and hunched over. A general depression settled like a murky fog over us all. But the nurses who weighed me and took my blood pressure would speak kindly to me. The doctor who met briefly with me and authorized the chemo radiated a hurried competency. Finally, I would be called to a numbered cubicle, and there would be Bill, energetic and quietly cheerful, wanting to know how I was doing as he gave me the anti-nausea pill and prepared the needle. I felt encouraged by his clothes, usually a broad-striped shirt and matching tie, and a white hospital coat with strips of bright orange, black, and green African cloth running up its lapels. We would talk like friends, glad to see each other, as he searched for a usable vein.

Sometimes the 5FU in the vial had just come from the refrigerator, and I felt its icy encroachment as it inched up the vein from my hand into my arm. Along with the 5FU I was given a drug called Levamisole in pill form, alternating weeks. Researchers had proven that Levamisole added to the 5FU greatly enhanced 5FU's effectiveness. It also, I soon discovered, made me very ill. And it had a curious history. "What it is," Bill explained one day, "is a de-worming agent for sheep and other farm animals. When it's used for sheep it costs six cents a pill." He raised his eyebrows, meeting my eyes. "A Dr. Moertel at the Mayo Clinic discovered that it could be used with human patients, but he was afraid they'd jack up the price. It was Johnson & Johnson that made Levamisole, so he went to them and told them he was gonna prescribe it for cancer patients and he got a promise from them that they would keep the price down. Next thing he knows, the price has gone up from six cents a pill to six *dollars* a pill."

As he spoke he had found a usable vein and inserted the needle. While the 5FU entered me, Bill continued, "So he gets mad. He goes to Johnson & Johnson and tells 'em he's gonna order the pills made for sheep and use them with his human patients." Bill shook his head. "But this was the Reagan era, so Johnson & Johnson went to the government and got them to pass a law forbidding the use of animal medicine in humans. So the price stayed just where they'd set it." As he withdrew the needle from my hand, Bill and my companion and I marveled at the cupidity of the drug companies, and our government's complicity.

Bill stroked my arm with his big warm hand before I left, urging me to eat more, as I had by then lost twenty pounds. "Ice cream!" he said. "This is your chance to pig out."

As I had thought of Deborah in the emergency room, I saw Bill as a bodhisattva, the Buddhist embodiment of compassion. In the midst of suffering and depression, he offered steady warm optimism. I wondered how he could maintain this stance—this reliable caring—day after day, year after year. Perhaps it was simply his willingness to do it that sustained him, for he did not seem to be guarding himself against the suffering he ministered to; and so there was no friction in the encounter. His fellow oncology nurse, Sally Walker, offered the same comfort. A white woman in her forties, she talked more than Bill, and would sometimes sit with her arm around me in the hallway, discussing my symptoms and promising to intercede with the doctor for me. She was always patient, always kind. These two I recognized as exceptional human beings, seemingly better able than the rest of us to tolerate stress and suffering, to move gracefully in what must have been a grueling work environment, and to offer kindness to everyone. In paintings of the Buddhist six realms of existence, in each realm, among animals, or hungry ghosts, or the sufferers in hell, there stands a bodhisattva, offering comfort and the possibility of enlightenment to the inhabitants of that realm. Sally and Bill echoed that image as they moved through the Oncology Clinic. I always looked forward to seeing them when I came for my treatment.

At home I lived with the side effects. While the loss of taste, fatigue, and other physical effects bothered me, the mental vagueness frightened me more. As if my mind had become a platform, certain items slid over to the edge and dropped off. One morning began with an errand, after which I locked my keys in the car, with the radio playing. In the parking lot of the drugstore, I got down on the concrete to crawl under my car, groping for the spare key that was wired to the underside of the wheel assembly. That same afternoon, in the warm bathroom, I was in the midst of an enema when the doorbell rang. "Who the hell is that?" I wondered. I pulled up my pants and went to the door, where I found one of my writing consultation clients. She handed me a card and some flowers from her garden. I thought, Well, she must be just dropping by to say hello. In the living room, we sat and chatted, though I had to run to the bathroom twice. Awkwardly I looked for a signal from the woman, who seemed to be waiting for something. Finally I said, "I have some work to do now."

She blinked at me. "Oh, aren't we going to go over my writing?"

In a flash, I remembered. We were to have a consultation at 1:00 P.M. Embarrassment flooded me. She was kind. "Well now I have an extra hour to do things," she told me, as if I had given her a gift, and she said she'd call to set up another appointment while I babbled about how *it's not like me* to make such mistakes.

Another time, near the end of my Saturday-afternoon Autobiography workshop, two women got up and said they had to leave. We finished, and a woman whose first time it was in the class asked, "Do you go until 5:30 every Saturday?" I looked at my watch and saw it was indeed 5:30—half an hour later than the class was supposed to end. Even though I had been looking at my watch, somehow I had not registered the time. I stammered, feeling exposed. One student said graciously, "I liked it; it was kind of like being allowed up after bedtime," and the others were casual about my mistake.

But after they left I felt shaken. Losing one's hair and one's sense of taste was one thing; losing one's mind was another. I felt unprotected, as if I were missing essential information. As if I might become incompetent at what I do. Oh, worst horror. Yet it was just details that were lost: my ability to teach the class and engage with the students remained fine, but selective peripheral information got lost. How could I deal with this?

Each morning I sat in communication with the dead mentors on my altar. Maurine Stuart regarded me challengingly; Lex Hixon smiled with unassuming gentleness; my parents wore their age with a kind of eagerness. My brother seemed very alive, looking out of his photograph. He had been eight years my senior, so that when I was a child he was already an adolescent, impatient with his little sisters. But sometimes when he and I were alone, he had gently teased me, looking at me with kind, caring eyes, and I had felt so happy to receive his attention. He had worked on jalopies in our driveway, a cigar stuck in the corner of his mouth, to the accompaniment of loud boogie woogie music rolling out of the phonograph—doing the things most calculated to infuriate my father. Beyond his adolescent unkindness to me and my sister, I never saw him be cruel to anyone. When my father harangued him at the dinner table, he only hung his head. Years after his suicide, when I was married and living in

San Francisco, he came to me in a dream and told me he had not died, that when he disappeared he had gone into the hills of West Virginia, where he was practicing with a spiritual teacher. In the dream we stood under trees outside his cabin; he wore a plaid wool shirt and his thick hair was gleaming in the sun, his dark eyes peaceful. I had awakened with tears streaming down my face.

Now I asked for my brother's help as I attempted to meditate. When I closed my eyes, sitting still in the relative silence of the living room, I could experience how the Levamisole veiled my mind, blurring areas of consciousness. At first I struggled against this, trying to maintain the focus of my meditation, but at moments I simply could not bring my attention to bear on my breath or other sensations. For some days I tensed in frustration, feeling this incapacity to meditate as a further insult. And then, as if my dead ones spoke to me, I understood the futility of my struggles, and that I was only increasing my suffering. Ruth Denison appeared in my mind, telling again the story of her disorientation, her fear that she was dying, and how she had been instructed to go ahead and die—that is, to surrender to what was actually happening rather than trying to avoid or manipulate it. Only when she did that could she pass through to a state of more balance. Finally I saw that I must give in to the vagueness, allow it, and gently observe it. As I began to relax, I found that while my mind did sometimes wander off into blurry side-trails, at other moments it came back, like a set of binoculars adjusting into sharp focus, and I was able to notice my breathing again.

Life with Crystal became a wild careening from light to dark. One day after she had accompanied me to chemo, I found her curled into a ball on the floor of her study, her face wet with tears. "Crystal, what's wrong?" I asked, alarmed at seeing her so helpless. I got down on the rug next to her, touched her shoulder. Gulping back tears, she told me, "It's like your illness takes up all the space in our relationship, you know? There's nothing left for me. My needs don't matter anymore. You're so self-absorbed you don't pay any attention to me." She began to cry again, and I held her. Stroking her hair, I felt my own helplessness. In the struggling to save my life, I did not have much energy left over to give to her. I felt guilty and sorry, as she said against my shoulder, "Sandy, I feel like I'm being pushed beyond my strength. I don't know how I can take this anymore."

Several days later, Crystal was her competent self who wanted to plan.

She understood that the coming months would be hard, and she wanted our communication to be better. We sat in a Chinese restaurant, and I choked down spoonfuls of wonton soup while she asked that each of us state our needs, so that we could both get at least some of what we wanted. "I don't feel very close to you right now," she said. "Your vitality is so low, it's as if I don't have anything to respond to. And you don't talk to me very much or tell me what you're feeling." I admitted that I did not have much strength to put into communicating with Crystal, as I was always exhausted. But as we talked over our egg rolls, it seemed possible to change—that I could appreciate her efforts more, could give her more support for the music class she was planning and remember to let her know if I was too tired to listen when she wanted to tell me about her life. I asked if we could try for more intimacy, since I missed the touching, and we agreed to try to move past the physical distance we had allowed to develop long before the cancer struck. Our discussion proceeded so rationally: it seemed we had made a workable plan, constructing a little boat to carry us through the rapids.

For hours each day I lay in bed, the bedroom shades drawn and the TV set silent. Sometimes I slept, sometimes I lay awake, letting my thoughts wander, searching for the source of a feeling I now had, that I had been radically altered—by the cancer, the surgery. I chased this awareness that hung just outside my grasp, and wound up each time puzzled. Talking about this quest would have been useless, I knew; for I understood that no one else could help me find the answer. The inkling followed me through the days until one night I awoke suddenly in the silent dark bedroom. Crystal lay turned away from me in the bed. I sat up, as if someone had called my name, and I recognized that something very deep inside me would never be the same as before. Perhaps it was a consciousness now available to me, of my death: the conviction of my own ultimate survival had been wiped away like condensation from a glass, and I could see into the truth of my coming disintegration. I sat staring into the darkness, electrified by this awareness. I knew that now I was living from a different center than before; the truth of impermanence was available to me now in a concrete way, in the very cells of my body.

As the days passed, I came upon new vulnerabilities. One Saturday afternoon three of the nine participants in my Autobiography class did not arrive. As the class started, my spirits sank. I felt distressed and shaky, thinking, "They don't like the workshop. I'm not a good teacher." While I taught the class, I struggled with my insecurities, which rumbled like an underground river. At the same time I wondered why I was taking it so hard, since I usually focused only on those who were present and did not worry about the absentees or their motives.

After class I listened to my phone messages: All three women had called, one sick, one with a crisis at home, and one with a celebration for her wedding anniversary. All my faltering and uncertainty had been without cause. I realized, once again, how we create our suffering. The Buddha taught that the identification with self leads to pain. It was my preoccupation with myself that had tripped me up: I had abandoned the requirements of the present moment, wondering, was I being sufficiently appreciated? was someone thinking ill of me?

We are slaves of praise and blame, the mind taking us away from the authentic experience of our lived moments. In my weakness I had fallen victim to this.

The weekly chemo visits became mini torture-sessions as my veins collapsed; the infusion could be accomplished only after multiple painful sticks with the needle. On Valentine's Day, Sandy Butler and I went to Highland and settled ourselves in the chaotic waiting room of the clinic. Near us sat three Middle Easterners, the woman in a black suit with a white scarf covering her hair. She looked to be in her fifties and had a sensitive face, her mouth pulled sideways from a stroke or seizure. Next to them, a tiny Hmong woman in a brown and yellow printed sarong sat with her two granddaughters. The grandmother's round lined face looked immensely cheerful; she seemed to be having a wonderful time. In front of us an African-American child who had come with her mother toddled about, clasping a little brown doll. She was maybe two years old, with a compact body, alert face, and pigtails sticking out to the sides. I saw how physically adept she was for being so small, as she negotiated chairs and large grown-up bodies. I glanced at her mother, a young woman who was gazing unhappily into space, and thought of all the young women suffering from cancer these days, the mothers of babies, who might not live to see their children grow up.

Sandy and I sat talking for the first couple of hours. "How's it going at home?" she asked. She also wanted to know how the drugs were affecting me, and whether I had started to plan for my birthday, which fell in the summer. Always, beneath our conversation, I was aware that Sandy knew the cancer-chemo routine intimately. Yet we rarely spoke about those three years in which her partner had fought to survive cancer, and then died of it.

The birthday question was not an idle one, for what Sandy liked most was to plan. She was, as she would put it herself, reflexively instrumental. Present her with any problem and she would go into strategy-mode, her mind listing and organizing and reaching for resources, and in a short while she would devise a plan of action. In the Wandering Menstruals meetings we teased Sandy about this ability when sometimes it seemed that she most loved planning *other* people's lives, whether they wanted her to or not. I knew that whatever else she might be feeling about my illness, she could get some satisfaction in taking command of the situation at various points.

Now as we sat in the Oncology Clinic, we continued our running conversation about our lives, and Sandy peered at the book on my lap.

"So what's that you're reading?" she asked.

I held up a book by Charlotte Delbo, called *Auschwitz and After.* "I've been trying to get through this but it's so harrowing! After each scene I have to recover."

"I can imagine," Sandy said. "You go for light reading these days, don't you, girl!"

Finally we were called into the inner sanctum, where a Dutch-born nurse named Gondica awaited us. Slim and bespectacled Gondica was always sympathetic. But I felt apprehensive, for she had never inserted the needle in me before, and I wondered how well she would negotiate my reluctant veins. Gondica greeted Sandy, whom I introduced—the nurses were intrigued by my arriving each week with a different person: "Who's your partner *this* week?" Bill would ask—then she sat me in a chair and gave me the anti-nausea pill. She noted the chemo burns on my right hand from last week and decided to use my left arm. After a painful stick in my arm, then one in my hand, from which each time the vein "rolled away," Gondica called for Bill Shanks. Bill arrived, looking hurried and concerned. I was momentarily relieved, until it became apparent that he too could not find a decent vein. He tried my right arm, but the vein he stuck eluded him. I sat with my arm out, Bill probing, Gondica hovering near, and Sandy sitting next to me murmuring to reassure me. For thirty minutes Bill tried this vein and that, poking and probing. The pain became hard to bear, and my frustration level rose. I breathed and tried to stay connected to my body, to reach a center of calm. To myself, I thought, "If it's going to be like this every week, I can't do it."

Finally Bill resorted to the hand already burned in an angry red-black patch by last week's chemo. He inserted the needle, and at last the clear fluid with the 5FU started to enter my vein. "Now you take it from here," Bill said to Gondica. With a squeeze of my arm, he left the cubicle.

How to contain the wild flutter of hysteria just beneath my mind? How to stay here with what had to be done? I began to tell Sandy about a scene in the Delbo book, and Gondica, still pushing the plunger on the syringe, said, "That happened to my brother." I asked her what she meant, eager to lift my focus from my painful hand. Gondica told how, during World War II, her nineteen-year-old brother had joined the underground in Holland to help the Jews escape. He could not live at home and had to be very circumspect in his comings and goings. Still, eventually he was betrayed, trapped in a house where there was no back door for him to escape. The Gestapo took him to jail and sent him to a concentration camp. "Did he ever return?" I asked.

Gondica carefully removed the needle from my hand and pressed a cotton ball over the entry point. "Later a man who had been in the camps with him came to my family. He said my brother had gotten sick with dysentery—the conditions in the camps were terrible—and he died." She pulled a strip of tape over the cotton and lifted my free hand to press my fingers on the tape, to stop any bleeding. "When the Allies came to liberate the camp," she continued, "the Germans put the prisoners on a boat and sent them to the middle of a deep lake, where they set the boat on fire, and all the prisoners burned or drowned. The man who came to us had been able to hide while this was going on, so he survived." She was sweeping away the clutter of used vials and cotton pads to make room for the next patient. I was absorbed in her story, imagining the family's shock. "How awful it must have been to hear the news!" Gondica waited a moment before replying, her eyes hooded. "Yes, it was a terrible blow."

When we left the hospital, Sandy put her arm around me. There was no time for grieving, for relaxing or recovering from this afternoon. I had to do some grocery shopping, cook dinner, and teach a workshop that evening. I carried Gondica's story in my heart, and connecting to that larger pain gave me strength, for it brought me a visceral awareness of the suffering of all humanity—in wars, in illness, in loss of loved ones, in death—that went on all over the world at all times; it revealed my own discomfort as merely another condition of being a human being, not exceptional or dramatic or to be avoided, and so made it easier to bear.

Like Crystal lying curled on the floor of her study, weeping, somewhere far back among the rooms of my serviceably furnished, fairly spacious, constructed self I lay hidden and hopeless, not weeping but stunned by a sense of helpless stillness in me. I was supported by many people: each of these generous ones came to help because they had known me during the thirty years I had lived here in the Bay Area and had been active and involved in public life; each of my helpers wanted to acknowledge that presence, to express affection or gratitude by her actions, for I had been part of a shared story. Now I participated in another story, the saga of cancer, of the epidemic among women, though for most it was breast cancer. This story was not created by me personally; it had been defined by others, some still alive, most of them gone, and it challenged, how can you step up to this, how can you meet it? In this story I found a way to play my part, allowing friends to help and appreciating them; engaging with the folks at Highland—nurses and patients alike—in order to situate my experience in normal life, to make it human-size and bearable. In return, my friends gave me their loving concern, their time and effort, and that felt palpably sustaining, as if a hundred strong hands lifted me.

But there was another, inner experience that could not be touched by that love. I would sit in the car next to a person driving me to my chemo appointment and know that I had sunk into that place of stillness—mute wondering, without hope. We did not know if the chemo would work. We did not know the end of the story. The words of a Buddhist teacher echoed in my head, positing that when we come to this awareness of our fundamental aloneness, we are on our way to discovering "a completely unfabricated state of being." I stayed with this opportunity for a time, and then I told myself a story. I said to myself, I am not dying, I have no intention of dying. But the story was not utterly convincing, for I knew it was possible that cancer cells had already reached my liver, or that a few still resided in my bowel. This not-knowing was the truth of my existence now, and as much as I communicated with others, it always pulled me back into aloneness. Buddhism is the path without hope; we are enjoined to go beyond hope and fear, and to simply be with our experience without interpretation, no matter what it may be. To live without certainties, without a guaranteed continuity or future, is the "unfabricated" condition. I did my best to stay faithful to this perception.

There is something inherently discouraging about allowing poison to be injected into one's veins, even for the greater good. It's a desperate measure, sacrificing one's (in my case) mucous membranes, one's energy, and sense of well-being in order to save the whole organism. This is the slash-and-burn modus operandi of the Western medical response to cancer. It's not unlike our military maneuvers, historically: go in and destroy everything—crops and forests, cities, transportation, water supply, women, men, and children—in hopes of getting the bad guys. I had agreed to accept this; now I had to live with the discomfort, my growing weakness, the loss of most of my hair (despite what they had told me), and the diminishment of my actual flesh. One day, leaning down to a car window on the sunny street, I had glimpsed my face reflected in the glass and had been stunned at the new spider web of lines circling my eyes and creasing my cheeks. This was an aged face, falling away from its former firm contours.

One evening I lay propped up in our bed, watching Crystal walk about the room, her eyes alternating between the TV set and the many papers spread across her side of the bed and encroaching on mine. She was so attractive to me, slender in green sweatpants, her hair springy as a pony's mane, her hands slim-fingered and refined in their movements. For the last few days she had been particularly busy, caught up in many tasks (some of them for my benefit), rarely finding a moment to be with me. Here in the room with her, wanting so much to be close to another human being—to be held and cherished—I felt a loneliness different from that helpless sinking back into myself where I encountered my essential aloneness. This had a familiar feel to it, perhaps a memory deep in my tissues of reaching out as an infant, a reaction to a denial of warmth.

And I was back in my childhood in the scrubby outskirts of Columbus, where we had to walk for a half a mile to and from school on a street without sidewalks, rain or shine or snow. In the schoolyard one morning recess, a great lake of a puddle had gathered from last night's rain. The bitter cold had frozen the puddle, and we children raced out on the ice to slide wildly about, screeching. As was my habit, I launched myself out farther than the other girls, vying with the boys in bold abandon.

The ice cracked under me, and suddenly I was floundering in icy water; I struggled upward, realizing that I was drenched to my thighs, my wool skirt hanging in dripping folds. Around me the others shrieked and strutted. I understood this was a crisis. Already my knees felt numb in the bitter cold air. It did not occur to me to go back into the schoolroom so that my teacher might help me; instead I left the schoolyard, crossed the highway where semi trucks roared, and started for home. I ran, panicked and colder than I had ever been in my life, my legs stinging and the wet skirt flopping against my thighs.

Past the old frame and shingle houses, the porches closed against winter, and the stripped black branches of the trees, I ran and then walked, my shoes squishing, then ran again, panting. I thought I would freeze to death before I reached home. When I came in sight of our stark white-framed house, I knew I would make it and ran again, pounding up the sagging wood steps.

My mother met me at the door, surprised to see me home, and assessed my condition. Upstairs she helped me take off my clothes, toweled off my legs, and put me into the bed I shared with my sister, pulling the covers up over my legs. I huddled under the bedclothes as they slowly warmed around me, shivering now uncontrollably, and gradually realized that I was safe.

My mother had left the room; soon she returned with a tray, on it the food we always got when we were sick: Campbell's chicken noodle soup and a stack of soda crackers. Gratefully I ate the greasy soup with its strong flavor of comfort. Then I lay back in the warm bed, warm finally myself, and began to feel a little of the trauma leave me. I would be safe here, I would not freeze in the awful hard cold air outside. Here in my room I had the bed all to myself, I could spread out and even take up some space on my sister's side. I felt coddled and soothed, and was drifting near to sleep when my mother came in again.

She picked up the tray, looking down at me, and said, "All right, now it's time to go back to school."

I was astonished. No way was I ready to leave this warm enclosure. Did she really imagine that I could go outside, walk in the icy air for half an hour, and enter the classroom again today? Her blue eyes confirmed that yes, she demanded this of me. I must resume my life immediately.

I lay in silent resistance. My sister and I did not dare to argue with our parents. But I wanted her to see by my stillness that this was not a workable plan—that I was not ready, not healed yet—not strong again.

"Get up and get dressed," she said, and left the room.

Twenty minutes later, I walked down the steps from the porch, wearing a dry skirt and my old pair of shoes that were too tight for me, and bundled in coat and wool hat. Inside I nursed a wintry outrage. Plodding in the bleak afternoon along the road, I longed for my warm bed, and could not imagine sitting in the classroom again among my peers. The walk in the cold dark afternoon became a purgatory, replete with messages.

My mother's truth: life goes on, and your feelings, weaknesses, and hurt draw away into insignificance before its requirements. No one cares how you feel about anything.

Now as I remember this I wonder, what does a child deserve? After all, my mother put me to bed, she fed me. Why was I convinced that I deserved more than that? Just as Crystal drove me to appointments, made lists, answered phone calls, and generally gave of her time and effort for me—why wasn't that enough? Was I a spoiled child then? Spoiled by my father's love for me, his letting me know I was his favorite, sheltering me and appreciating me? I knew I was precious to him, and that made me precious to myself, made me imagine that I deserved comfort and healing. My daddy was a person of extremes, wholehearted in his love and fiery in his rages, committed to bitterness and judgment, moved by a great well of sweetness in him, unpredictable and sometimes scary. He was out of control, more like a big dangerous child than a grownup.

My mother's strict Scottish, New England economy extended to her emotional life. Once, after she died, I sat in the graveyard sobbing for her, broken open by my awareness of the limitations ingrained in her, and by her larger self, the passionate, powerful woman who never became real in the world, as if this possibility had hovered ghostlike behind her strictly controlled, respectable persona—the erect redhead in the navy blue suit and gold button earrings—whose only sins were those of omission.

I had participated in causing Crystal's emotional disappearance long before the cancer came to toss our lives in the air. Now and then, in frustration, I had acted out my father's rage, brutally slamming a door while

I yelled or throwing something, and that wild anger had frightened Crystal. She began the dance of withdrawal that was so habitual to her that she was not even conscious she was doing it. I know I was partly to blame, and that in some ways it served me to live a life in proximity but not in deep contact. Maybe it felt familiar, like having a mom who dressed and fed me but almost never held me close, never yelled at me, and never shed tears for me or in front of me. Maybe I secretly preferred the distance to the messy tangle of a shared emotional life. When we were first together and Crystal would insist on participating in some activity with me, occasionally I would think to myself, "Too much *with*."

Now I sat in the bed, my head down, and realized that the "with" had disappeared long before. Had I trusted her more, or had I been less well defended, I might have let Crystal see my devastation. If she could have glimpsed my utter vulnerability, there might have been a chance that she could have softened, truly wanted to understand, and entered with me into my experience of this illness.

But the chemo had brought me to my knees. Literally I felt as if I knelt, my head bent and my body curled over itself to protect what strength I had left. I did not have the energy to initiate any kind of process to change things. That gesture was beyond my strength.

Sitting in the bed watching Crystal move about the room, shuffle papers, and make notes, all the while glancing at the television screen, I wondered, What is the truth in this muddle of concepts, feelings, history? I was left confused and wounded, feeling a huge wistful longing for what I wished could be there.

13

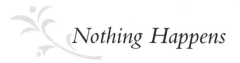

Nothing Happens

All changes at a blow
Springs of water welling from the fire.
Kaso Sodon

ONE MONTH after starting the chemotherapy, I began the writing of
Opening the Lotus. Unlike previous books, which had required my inter-
viewing many people, gathering information, transcribing tapes, reading
source material, and evoking and synthesizing others' views, this book
required me simply to draw upon my fifteen years of Buddhist practice
and study and tell what I knew. It was the perfect task, for now, in my
state of diminished energy, I could not have gone out into the world to
gather material.

Each morning for three to four hours I sat at my desk and worked on
the book. No matter how I felt, I went into my study and began where
I had left off the day before. The writing became a time of healing for me.
Sitting at my desk, I was not a cancer patient, a sick person, a disem-
powered and gravely threatened person. I left that behind and entered the
task fully; I became my action, and in this I was empowered.

That was a great teaching: that no matter how sick we may be, there
is always a dimension of us that is intact and healthy. Whether through
creative work, through sensitive contact with others, through spiritual
practice, or through appreciation of music or art, we can at moments
access that other reality. Perhaps it is the same place I touched when I
called upon Kwan Yin in the graveyard.

Three months had passed since I had communicated with the circle of
people who were helping me through this illness. Now, in another letter,
I told them:

It's a treat when someone comes over to help with something, and we have a visit at the same time. Lenore and I talked about this when she came to take me on a shopping trip. We had such a good time doing this chore together that we talked about the concept of "barn-raising and corn-shucking." In the early days of this country that's how people socialized. One family needed help with the harvest. Everyone came to help, did the work and then ate and drank and had a good visit. That's the kind of getting together I'm experiencing. Lenore and I talked about how interesting it would be to combine work and visiting even when we're able-bodied, to go help someone scrub her floor or work in her yard and then sit down to drink tea or have a meal. In this way we would come to know each other differently, experiencing the texture of each other's lives and participating in some of the essential labor.

Each morning I meditate at my altar. Recently I felt my heart blossoming like a lovely white flower. And I realized that Lex Hixon had been teasing me when he said I'd have to keep my center all year to earn this flower in my heart. I have it now—delicate, gleaming—perhaps not radiating light as much as his, but that will come. The joke's on me, Lex's making it seem the flower would be the result of effort, when it's simply there.

I was helped at times, oddly enough, by ruminations on death, shared with a group of people in a church basement in Berkeley. I found this support group through a Buddhist friend, Rick Fields, editor of the *Yoga Journal* and author of *How the Swans Came to the Lake*, the definitive book on Buddhism's arrival and establishment in the United States. Rick, who had been struggling with metastatic lung cancer for a year, took me to his group. On my first visit, I found myself shy and hesitant, uncertain whether I could talk to strangers about my disease. The leader, a nurse named Jan, was busy setting up chairs in a circle in the small, cold room, but she took time to smile and welcome me. When the chairs had filled with people, because I was new they introduced themselves: Marsha, a therapist, who had been dealing for several years with breast cancer; Rick Kohn, a man in his mid forties with a shock of brown hair and a sweet smile (I realized I had met him briefly, years before; he was a scholar of Tibetan Buddhism, afflicted now with bladder cancer); Joyce, a young woman who sat with her husband on the couch, herself a victim of advanced breast cancer. Several older women spoke of their lung cancer.

Then Jan set up a little bell in the center of the circle and asked us to be silent for a moment and listen while she rang it. I knew that Rick Fields had suggested the bell and brought it, offering a spiritual touchstone for the group. Now, with me here, there would be three Buddhists attending.

Jan rang the bell and we sat in silence as the vibrations faded.

Then people began to talk, sharing information and giving each other moral support. Gradually I relaxed. Often someone laughed, grimly amused by the surreal world of cancer treatment. Now and then someone spoke out angrily; once, Rick Kohn's eyes filled with tears. When the meeting ended, I knew I wanted to come to the next one.

For months I arrived every other Friday morning at the church and helped Jan set up the chairs. I came to know the people, tracking their treatment with them, and opening to their feelings. The group became very important to me, for here was a place where explanations were not necessary, where I could talk about a proposed treatment and hear, from people who had experienced it, what it felt like to receive it. Doctors always minimized the effects of any procedure or drug; my friends in the support group gave me the truth. And we laughed a lot. Sometimes when things get too bad, they get funny. We would guffaw over the non-choices offered to cancer patients. "Well, you can do this horrific treatment or you can do this other even more grotesque one. Of course neither of them may work. Now which would you prefer?" We giggled about the "side" effects of treatments and made bitter jokes about the sometimes appalling attitudes of doctors and other caregivers. The most egregious insults and instances of medical incompetence made us chortle. Being among these people was wonderfully restorative.

After some meetings I would join Rick Fields and Rick Kohn at lunch in a Jewish deli or a sushi place. Now and then we talked about how it felt to be the resident Buddhists in the group, with the leader sometimes deferring to us as though because we meditated, we possessed some secret about how to meet our cancer. Rick Kohn grinned. "What do *we* know?" And Rick Fields answered, "All we know is that we don't know. Maybe the thing practice has given us is just to be aware of what we're doing—whether we can change it or not." But we agreed that there was perhaps something useful we brought to the group from our Buddhist perspective, for even when we had been most healthy, we had been asked to contemplate our own disintegration, to allow for the passing away of everything we knew and held dear, and to accept this impermanence as a natural part of living. In Tibetan Buddhism there are practices designed to prepare one for death; *The Tibetan Book of the Dead*, made famous by the hippies, details this system. In Theravada Buddhism, an advanced practice, done only by Asian meditators as far as I know, consists in watching the gradual decay of a human corpse; at the front of the meditation hall in the nunnery in Sri Lanka where I had meditated hung a skeleton. Perhaps Rick Fields, Rick Kohn, and I were more at home with ideas of disintegration and death than the others, and that perspective could be a balancing factor in the group.

One morning, gathered in the church basement, our group found ourselves talking about a member who was in the process of dying. Joyce, lying against pillows on the couch, told about Marjorie, a woman whom I had met only once. Marjorie had arranged with her family that when it was clear she was at the point of death, they would put her in their van and drive out to a park. With her family around her, under the trees, in the open air, Marjorie would say her goodbyes. Her husband's brother, a physician, would give her a lethal injection, and she would die.

We sat pondering the story. People talked, appreciating Marjorie, who had been an accomplished and witty woman, saying they felt her presence with us. Several people cried. The illegality of this death, a fact of no importance, was not mentioned.

Then Rick Fields described a retreat he had just attended, on the dying process as it is viewed in the Tibetan Buddhist tradition. Rick was a short man in his fifties, with a lively expression and bright, interested eyes. He always wore blue jeans and a casual shirt, and sometimes covered his nearly bald head with a baseball cap. His voice scratched in his throat as he talked. He told about how the *bardo,* or "in-between state," is present in our lives so much, that we die with each outbreath. Then he admitted his anxiety after being with one of our members as she was dying: how she had been "floating" on morphine, a little out of touch. Rick wanted to *be there* when he died, fully conscious until the last moment. He asked the lamas about this and they said it didn't matter—that at death both the physical being and the mental self are disintegrating, but the essence cannot be touched and does not change. In other words, "nothing happens." So whether one is drugged on morphine in the midst of this disintegration or not is not important. "He told me to relax and take any pain medications I needed," Rick said, giving a broad relieved smile.

This talking about death felt so right. We were like little children going into a realm that we couldn't understand—at times fascinated, then scared, then angry or depressed, and then fascinated again.

Joyce was in bad shape. She lay back against the couch, her legs on her husband's lap, and fiddled with the tube connecting her to the squat canister of her portable oxygen tank. Joyce always managed to look rakish, her bald head covered by a silken, richly dyed turban, her body draped in loose, stylish clothes. As usual, she spoke with a sort of astonishment, as if asking, Can it really *be* this way, or am I about to wake up? Now she told us that the pain in her back from the metastasis had been nearly uncontrollable during the preceding week.

Her husband, a tall, vigorous man with the same unbelieving look that Joyce wore, cupped his hands on her knees, holding her legs against him, and told how the combination of chemotherapy and pain killers had sent her into a week of "Olympic vomiting—I thought she'd burst her rib cage if she didn't stop." They looked much too young for this terminal suffering, like people just starting out on the long shared life that they should have had. I watched them, feeling at once sad for them and envious of their closeness.

"I decided it was time to die," Joyce said, "and I almost made the decision to do it. Now I feel better." She smiled ironically. "Before, the disease didn't cause me pain: the treatments did. Now the cancer *and* the treatments are both unbearable. I didn't want to go on. And I thought, 'I'm a wimp. I'm giving in.'" Her husband said the week had been important for her family—to see her that way, to accept that she might choose to die rather than suffer that much.

A new group member talked. She was plump and baldheaded, with recently diagnosed metastatic breast cancer. "A death sentence," she said. She was going to have a bone marrow transplant soon, and it was her only chance. Her husband sat next to her, withdrawn and uncommunicative. She said that his way of coping was to work too hard, his job taking him away from home most of the time. I thought of Crystal's distance, her disappearance into her preparation for the class.

Before I left, I hugged Joyce and Rick, clinging to their warm, fragile bodies. What was it that had been so grounding, so reassuring, in this discussion? Perhaps it was to be drawn into the reality of death in life, of the darkness in the light. I thought, again, of the Zen teacher Joko Beck's metaphor of the little whirlpools in a stream. Defined for a time, the whirlpool has its own contours, width and depth and movement, and yet it is not separate from the flowing water of the stream. Just so, our individual lives hold their contours for a while, create their own identities. Then they break up and disintegrate out into the flow. We call this death, and feel like something momentous has happened; and yet, seen from another perspective, the stream merely continues its flow, and "nothing happens." That is, while believing in our whirlpool, we have nevertheless been part of the stream. It is possible for us to know both realities, both the shape of our separate lives and the timeless flow of energy that is our enduring reality. Joyce and Rick, and the absent Marjorie, had brought me to this experience, even if only for that morning.

I drove home from the meeting feeling the expansion of this wider awareness.

As the weeks of chemotherapy wore on, I became more and more ill. Weakness took me, until I could barely stand upright, and had to take several naps a day. My sense of taste deserted me, leaving only one flavor, which was like sawdust laced with chemicals. I lost weight steadily. There were only certain foods I could get down, a very narrow range: hot cereal, African food, burritos. Then, one day, eating in the Asmara, the Eritrean restaurant around the corner from our house, I felt my throat close, gorge rising, and I knew I would no longer be able to eat this food. The burritos were next to go. My eyes hurt so much I could barely read; the skin on my fingers cracked and bled.

Economics intruded as well. My alternative supplements and herbs cost about three hundred dollars a month, so my expenses had swelled; at the same time, my income went down, since I did not have the strength to do private writing consultation or editing to supplement what I earned from classes and publishing. Sandy Butler took me out for tea. As we sat across the table from each other in a noisy bakery, she pulled a legal pad out of her tote bag and fixed me with an imperious gaze.

"I want you to tell me every one of your expenses, and I'm going to make a list."

"But why?" I asked, reluctant to dwell on the subject of my depleted finances.

"Never mind, just tell me."

Silently I looked at her.

"It's so we can make a plan, dummy. Now, come on."

I obeyed, mentioning amounts for rent and utilities, food, supplements, and Chinese herbs, as she wrote them down.

Sandy made quick calculations. "Now here's the total. And these days how much do you make in a month?"

I answered, and she shook her head.

"Not so good. Hmm. So okay, here's what we're going to do. I'll write a letter to some people in the community who might be wondering how they can help. When I suggest it to them, they may want to send you some amount monthly toward your support while you're doing the chemo."

I drew back. "Oh…I don't think I can do that."

She pierced me with a reproving stare. "Sandy, stop yourself right now. You want to make it through this hard time, don't you?"

"Yes."

"And it's true that you can't earn enough money to meet your expenses."

"Yes."

"All right then. Do you really want to spend the whole time worrying and going into debt?"

My heart had begun to beat rapidly. I felt lightheaded. "This is hard for me," I told her. "It would feel like begging."

Sandy leaned toward me. "Answer me this. If one of your friends was in trouble and needed money to survive, would you send some?"

"Yes."

"And would you think less of her because she was in trouble?"

"No."

She sat back, meeting my eyes with a steady gaze. "Okay." Sandy lifted her tea cup and took a sip. She tapped the legal pad on the table between us. "Now, *you* don't have to send out the letter. I will write it and send it, on your behalf, and the money can be sent to me to be put into a fund for you. Then each month I'll just give you any checks I receive."

"Really?"

"Yes, girl, trust me that there are people in this community who want to see you make it through this and get well, and they'll be happy to help you do that."

Sandy was right. In response to her letter a number of people donated monthly. Because she had told them any amount would be greatly appreciated, some people responded with small checks, some with large; and the fund thus created allowed me to meet my expenses.

Near the end of April, a milestone was passed. My veins had completely failed, and would no longer accept the needle. Sally Walker, oncology nurse, reminded Dr. Cutting, head of Oncology, that what needed to be done for me now was the insertion of a "portocath." This is a device surgically inserted in one's chest, with a catheter going into the vena cava above the heart. Chemicals can be injected by needle into the Portocath and they go directly into the system, traveling through the body in the blood flow.

No way did I want to endure another surgery, but my support group assured me that the Portocath would relieve me of much suffering. "You'll never have to be poked fifteen times in the hand again!" Joyce told me. "Look here!" Rick Fields said, pulling open his shirt to show me the lump under his skin just below his collar bone. "It's really no big deal." So finally I said yes.

At the hospital just before the surgery, while I lay waiting to be taken into the operating room, I read a piece in the Buddhist paper *Turning Wheel*. It was an interview with Sister Chan Khong, who works with the renowned Vietnamese monk Thich Nhat Hanh. The interviewer asked how Chan Khong confronted despair. "It is a matter of survival," she answered. "Everyone is capable of serenity when nothing difficult is before them. But when there are bombs dropping, you can be overcome by fear and hatred. When our friends were murdered doing social service in Vietnam, we did our best to calm ourselves. We saw that in order to survive we had to walk in the direction of beauty."

She spoke of the boat people escaping Vietnam, who were adrift on the high seas and menaced by pirates. She had rented a boat in Thailand, disguised herself as a fisherman, and "went out to sea to 'fish' out the boat people." During this time she was fearless and joyful, she said, even when faced with pirates, because she understood the rightness of her actions.

At the end of the interview Sister Chan Khong described some of the challenges of living at Plum Village, the community established by Thich Nhat Hanh in France. I knew people who had gone to France to visit this haven for short periods. I lay in the hospital bed thinking about Sister Chan Khong's dangerous life during the Vietnamese War and afterward, her indomitable spirit, and her commitment to nonviolence.

Finally the nurses wheeled me into surgery, a doctor gave me a sedative, and after a few moments I went off to Plum Village. For the next hour I watched children playing happily in the sunlight, walked among adults working in beautiful gardens, and saw people loving and supporting each other. I had some vague notion that someone was doing something on my chest, but that did not distract me from my visit. When I woke up, I had a wound, and under it a lump like a hard marshmallow pushing up the skin of my chest just below my left collarbone: the Portocath was in place.

14

Give Yourself to the Desert

*The point is still to lean toward the discomfort of life and see
it clearly rather than to protect ourselves from it.*

Pema Chodron

HOW STRANGE IT WAS to arrive at Dhamma Dena on an airplane, when
I was so used to the grueling ten-hour drive down Route 5 through the
San Fernando Valley. At the Palm Springs airport I was met by one of the
residents of Dhamma Dena, who lives in a small house near the meditation hall. Margaret bundled me into her car and drove out through the
desert toward the town of Joshua Tree while I gazed into the sunstruck
landscape, where yuccas spiked up from the dry earth and distant hills lay
like piles of children's blocks.

At Dhamma Dena, they put me in a room by myself in the recently
acquired Samadhi House, a short walk from the eating hall. I had never
before had the luxury of staying alone at Dhamma Dena. Here was offi-
cial recognition that I was ill, and I responded with ambivalence. On the
one hand I wanted to blend into the retreat, to be just another sitter,
another pair of hands for chores. In the eating hall, a stuffed parrot hung
from the ceiling, and from its golden beak dangled a card that read, "We
are in training to be nobody special." I had often repeated this to myself,
working against my need for achievement and recognition, and the dis-
content that it could engender. "I am in training to be nobody special."
Saying the words in my mind, I felt how they redirected me from a certain seductive struggle, excitement, and dis-ease into a more stable focus:
forget what others think of you, forget the future goal of achievement.
Arrive instead in this body and mind, attending to this present moment.
This is the whole of practice.

So I felt some discomfort at being set apart from the other women (This was the spring all-women retreat) and given a privilege. On the other hand, I was glad not to have to share this spare, light-filled room, grateful that the second single bed would remain unoccupied. Although the week would be passed in silence, precluding conversation with a roommate, still the presence of another human being would have required an output of energy, even if only to work out the essential logistics: when would the light be turned out at night? who would get which drawer in the bureau? and so forth. I knew that my capacity to negotiate was extremely diminished.

I hung my clothes in the small closet and sat down on the bed, letting myself become aware of the silence. At home in our house in Oakland, I lived with the dull under-roar of freeway and rapid-transit noise. Here in the desert the silence opened wide, the air so empty of sound that the buzz of a distant motorbike could stun the ear, making an obscene trail through the aural landscape until it fell away and the silence closed again. Looking out the window I saw a tall, spindly-armed creosote bush, its branches adorned with yellow blossoms, dancing in the wind. It bobbed and tossed, reached out, pulled back. I knew that the creosote was an ancient plant that had lived in this desert long before humans came. It was exquisitely adapted to its dry environment, able to live for years without water. Its deep roots in time and its ability to endure made the creosote a comfort for me to see.

Farther out in the desert stood a white house-trailer. In the last ten years Ruth had acquired several trailers to supplement the sleeping space for retreats. Each time she brought in a new trailer, she organized a work crew of meditators to clean it up. Smiling, I remembered the task of working on one particular trailer when it had first arrived back in 1984 or so. We had spent a long hot afternoon ripping up the filthy, sand-encrusted carpet. Then Ruth led us in the scrubbing of the walls. It had been hard, dirty, sweaty work.

Sometimes in her Dharma talks Ruth would describe the ways in which she had created the complex of buildings that was now Dhamma Dena. The main house had been a one-bedroom cottage before the addition of the dining room, and its kitchen had been extremely small. Ruth asked a student from Canada who was a builder to come down to add on a new kitchen, which Ruth's husband Henry had designed. The shelves in the kitchen were scavenged from a fabric store in Los Angeles. (Most of the materials in the buildings here were "harvested," as Ruth put it, from the desert or picked up in Los Angeles—on trash-collection night in wealthy Beverly Hills, for example.)

Ruth also told about her nearest neighbor, teaching us the Buddhist practice of "skillful means," in which a potentially obstructive person was transformed into a friend and advocate. Skillful means requires an awareness of the larger environment surrounding any situation, an assessment of all the forces at work there, and an appreciation for the needs of all the participants. The goal is always to promote the well-being of everyone concerned. In employing skillful means, one cannot close up and resist; always one moves toward engaging with the situation to find a solution.

This neighbor often worked in the yard, a short square man bending over the engine of a car. We had heard his voice many times, raised in impatience as he corrected one of his children. "Yes, I think he had the capacity for brutality," Ruth said, "but he was also very beautiful." Whenever there was a celebration or special meal at a retreat, Ruth had invited the neighbor and his family to come, and sometimes they did. When he had been putting a roof on his house, Ruth sent people from the retreat to help him, and they finished the job in a few hours. When she wanted to build a fence between the two houses, she baked a chocolate cake and went to have a talk with the neighbors with it in hand. "How do you feel about this," she asked them, "that we put up this fence so we don't disturb you?" Later her neighbor brought her more than a third of the lumber for the fence.

One day in the meditation hall, as she spoke of the labor of creating and maintaining Dhamma Dena, Ruth said, "*Life* is the practice, do you see? I don't feel disturbed by going out and working at this and taking care of that. I invite everybody else to participate, to really *see* how our practice works in action, hmm? So when you are working in the trailer you are practicing, just as when you clean your own home you can be practicing. Otherwise there is the temptation to tune into these wonderful *ideas* about Buddhism or enlightenment. You have to see that the ideas get tied into the reality behind them. It's nothing special. I have always done it. I don't even do it out of determination to show you; it's just natural for me to be there and to let it unfold together. It's really the best teaching."

I awoke to twilight outside the window, and struggled up from the exhausted sleep that took me, now, several times each day. Looking around the room, I realized how much change and flow had happened at Dhamma Dena since those early years of building. This Samadhi House in which I lay had been the neighbor's residence. He and his family had left the desert several years before, selling their low stone house to Ruth, and she had turned it into a dwelling place for female retreatants. She had christened it *"samadhi,"* meaning concentration or a deep meditative state. And perhaps its name said something about Ruth's gradual mellowing over time, for the first women's house, a few minutes' walk down the dirt road, was called Dukkha House.

When we were first coming here to the desert—a ragtag band of young hippies, political activists, and fledgling healers in the early eighties—Ruth had emphasized *dukkha*, the Buddha's First Noble Truth, the truth of suffering that was embedded in each moment of our human lives. Now, so many years later, my body filled with deadly chemicals and my energy burning low, I had more intimate knowledge of this great truth.

I pushed myself up from my bed and looked at my watch to see that the evening meditation would begin in half an hour.

Out in the fresh desert wind, I walked past the lighted windows of the dining hall, where women were finishing the last of the evening meal clean-up. Unlike them, I would have no chores during this retreat. Signing in, earlier, I had acceded to the manager who told me, "Ruth says not to give you a chore. She says to save your strength for meditating."

Walking in the dusk among the bobbing creosote and sage bushes, I felt my fragility, and breathed deeply of the cool clear air. Out here in the desert near the meditation hall, some other women had arrived early and were gazing at the horizon. We lingered, looking up at the low clouds that spread out like a sweep of white canvas from the horizon. Soon this pure expanse exploded with purple, orange, and golden light. We stood in silence under the wind, dark motionless figures among the chaparral, and the magnificent sweep of color was like the roof of a tent over us, growing paler at its boundaries inch by inch. There came a roar, approaching, filling the sky. I looked up, seeing nothing for a time. Then, far above the grandiose cape of color, in a sky of blue-black brilliance, I saw the flashing lights of a fighter jet, two red and one white. The jet made a heart-lifting curve and headed toward the first pale star. Now I saw behind the first jet another, with green eyes blinking. The jets streaked forward in that great hum of sound, passed under the star, and were gone.

In the meditation hall I positioned myself so that I could lean against the wall if necessary, and sat down on my pillow. I watched the women enter, twenty-five or so of them, and take their seats. These were not the scruffy rebels of previous times but mature-looking women, some wearing long skirts and colorful shawls. Perhaps we had simply grown up. At the front of the room, on a low platform, a bronze statue of the Buddha sat before a large mosaic disk. To his left stood a white-ceramic Kwan Yin, her eyes lowered in meditation, one hand lifted in the gesture of protection.

Someone rang the bell and the meditation began, silence deepening in the room. I closed my eyes, straightened my back, arranged my crossed legs, and clasped my hands before me. But soon I found myself sagging. This posture that was so familiar to me seemed to have lost its stability and my body had to struggle to maintain it. I straightened my curving back, lifted my chin, resolved to be erect and present. The minutes passed, falling away into the stillness. I brought my attention to my breath, but my senses seemed muffled and distant. The weakness gathered in me again, pulling my shoulders forward, weighting my head. Again I willed myself to sit up straight.

A voice spoke softly immediately before me, so close it startled me. "You are straining."

I opened my eyes and saw Ruth squatting before me, her rose-colored skirt falling in folds from her knees, her forehead creased with concern. Gently she reached forward to touch my shoulders.

"You don't need to sit up. Here, let me help you."

At first I felt only confusion. How could Ruth, so often stern where illness was concerned, suggest that I might lie down? And in the meditation hall!

But she guided me with her hands, and I surrendered to the relief of abandoning my upright position. Gently, Ruth lay me down on my back, placing a pillow under my head and pulling a shawl up over my body. So it was true; she was giving me permission to lie down during the meditation!

Often in the years before, I had seen her urge others to make effort even if they were ill. Now I did not know how to interpret her kindness, but could only receive it, realizing as I relaxed into the floor that indeed I was not *able* to sit like the others, no matter how I willed myself to do it.

Ruth stayed next to me for a few moments before moving on, her hand warm on my shoulder, as if convincing me by her touch that it was all right to give in to my weakness. The meditation continued as I lay with eyes closed, letting myself be aware of my reclining posture, gratefully visiting my back and legs, and my head supported by the pillow.

The next morning, I settled in to the retreat. I had forgotten how pleasant the women's retreats could be. For the last couple of years I had come down to the holiday retreat over New Year's, which was a rougher experience, crowded with more people, both men and women, and taking place in sometimes rainy or even snowy cold weather. At this retreat, in the meditation hall and eating hall, a gentleness reigned. The women, most of whom I had never met, seemed intelligent and sensitive, diligent in their practice and receptive to Ruth's instructions.

But I did not like being the one who had to lie down in the meditation hall. It made me realize how attached I was to the idea of myself as strong and energetic, seeing mind-pictures of myself at former retreats striding briskly across the desert, sitting steadfastly, scrubbing the shower room. The past made a cruel comparison.

On the second morning, during the early sitting, wrapped in a shawl in the dim light of the meditation hall, I was flooded suddenly with an exhaustion more total than anything I had yet experienced. And with it came a bottomless sadness. I left the meditation hall to walk back to my room, and curled up in my bed, the tiredness weighing like lead in my body. I realized that perhaps I had been holding myself together at home with considerable effort, manufacturing energy so that I could write *Opening the Lotus*, teach my classes, and get to my chemo appointments. This posture had seemed necessary at home; now I wondered about my need to think of myself as someone who could function well no matter what the conditions. "You are straining," Ruth had said. And I knew that in Buddhist practice one is asked to make strong effort but never to push in a self-punishing way. Perhaps, in the last months at home, I had been drawing from an empty well of illusory strength. Here in my room at Dhamma Dena, where there were no requirements to meet, my body let go, sinking down to the depth of my actual fatigue. I cried, feeling sorry for myself for having cancer. I cried also because I was ashamed of having cancer. Secretly I had nurtured the idea that only losers get this disease—or repressed people—or people who haven't done their emotional work. To protect myself from the possibility, I had told myself it was *those others* who were susceptible, not I who had always been the strong one, the brave one, the bold one. Now I had joined the ranks of the disabled, and it was hard for me.

Even though Ruth had given me permission not to follow the schedule of the retreat, I felt ashamed that I could not come to every sitting, could not do my "yogi" job. On previous retreats, I had judged people who did not meet the challenge. Now that I could not meet it, all my concepts and ideas, all my requirements about how people should be, rose up to taunt me. I castigated myself: during those years of doing Buddhist practice, trying to pierce to a deeper reality, still I had secretly held to my petty judgments. Defending the self, solidifying the self.

Lying in bed, staring across at the elaborate fluted lampshade of a ceramic lamp that had probably been picked up at a sidewalk trash-removal site, I thought about how cancer used to be: when I was young, people who got cancer just died, in more or less time. Now if you were lucky you could live, but you had to fight: do the chemotherapy and other therapies, do the complementary care, take care of yourself, go to a support group, do your spiritual practice. How exhausting! You had to *want* to live. Because I wanted to live I had to keep going, to carry this great weight of sadness in me, and sink under the shame.

Beginning to cry again, I felt that I no longer wanted to fight. I was too tired to struggle anymore.

All morning I stayed in bed, sleeping and crying, then sleeping some more.

At lunch, to which I had come shakily, Ruth entered the dining hall and asked for volunteers for a small project. She wanted some of us to sew loops on the kitchen rags in order to make them easier to hang up. What a picayune project this was, I thought, how very detail-oriented and Germanic of Ruth to think up such a thing! But to my surprise, I found myself raising my hand to volunteer.

After lunch, four of us met on the concrete porch next to the kitchen. We pulled up metal chairs to a little spool table piled with rags. The blazing midday sun beat down on the roof above us; at the end of the porch a woman washed the cooking pots at the outside sink. From my companions' smiles, I could see that they too found this task somewhat whimsical.

We cut small loops of cloth, folded them, and began to sew them to the corners of the rags. Gradually we began to take our task seriously, threading needles, shaping the loops. I felt the faintest of breezes against my bare arms. Colored cloths, hands lifting, lowered eyes, all of us gently together. My enormous vulnerability was safely cradled in this little circle of women. Finishing the first one, a woman held up the cloth with a loop affixed at its corner. "Is this how it's supposed to look?" she whispered, glancing about to make sure only we heard her, for this was a silent retreat. Someone grinned, and whispered back, "If Ruth came by she'd probably tell you to do it differently." We chuckled in knowing amusement. Then we returned into our silent task.

Held in that little circle, so much a part of these women and so involved in this simple chore, I felt the morning's sorrow gradually subside in me.

The next day, during the hours alone in my room, I could think of nothing but Crystal and our difficulties. I understood that she was in a state of serious panic: panic about my cancer, unacknowledged; panic about preparing for the class she would teach; panic about being able to earn a living; panic about her responsibilities as a homeowner and landlady. I wanted to support her in her efforts, and I wanted to be able to tend to the tasks of my own healing too. What was the "right understanding" of our predicament? I wondered, going for guidance to the Buddha's Eightfold Noble Path. That would require assessing how my own behavior tended to create more pain and conflict, and what might lessen the intensity of the negative feelings. Certainly, harsh language did not help—when I reacted with anger or sarcasm to something Crystal did. Then, also, was there some dishonesty going on, and selfishness? In my determination to soldier on, no matter how I felt, I was not letting Crystal see my weakness, so while I longed for her sympathy, perhaps I was preventing her from giving it.

But most damaging of all were the expectations I held—that Crystal could be emotionally nurturing, loyal, and generous even at the expense of her own needs. I had the inkling, even as I was imprisoned in these expectations, that another reality existed, that perhaps if I were able to see

Crystal simply as she was and not as I wanted her to be, I might feel her love for me and be able to express mine for her. It seemed that, rather than asking her to change, I needed to alter my own behavior and expectations of our relationship, to let go of some of my assumptions about how we should be together.

I sat on the floor in my little room under the fluffy lampshade, writing in my journal and pondering what I could step away from. Buddhism is the path of renunciation. We are taught to let go of our resistance to things. As Pema Chodron says, "The goal of renunciation is realizing that we already have exactly what we need, that what we have already is good." If I could renounce my expectations of my life with Crystal, perhaps I could experience what energy and warmth and goodness was there behind it all.

So I made a list:

1) I must let go of the desire that Crystal be other than she is. 2) I must stop expecting her to be open to me emotionally, and I must try to share with her more of what is going on with me. 3) I must give up my anger at her for her demands on me around money and housework. 4) I must not keep hoping to resume a sexual relationship.

Looking at my list, I decided that we could go on living as before, but without the expectations. We could take "time out" until I finished the chemo, living in a sort of marriage of convenience until then. Without expectations, if Crystal were kind to me, I could receive it in the moment, enjoy it and let it go. If she were unkind, the same.

I mapped out what I could do to support Crystal and help her, and what I was not able to do. I vowed not to expect Crystal to help me with my "cancer project" unless she specifically offered. If necessary, I would find other people to take me to the hospital for further treatment or surgery if I became ill. I would not expect Crystal to take care of me unless she offered. I would not expect her to share emotionally with me in this journey.

I understood that I was seeking to create and maintain a peaceful psychic, emotional environment in which healing could take place. What was at stake in the next eight months of chemotherapy, I knew, was my very life. If I did this well, I might never have a recurrence and might live to a ripe old age. If I did it badly and had a recurrence, I might always wonder if the emotional and psychic hassle interfered with my fully receiving the benefits of the chemotherapy. Our recurrent wrangling about money and the house had begun to feel literally poisonous to me, as if a toxic miasma rose from the floor under me.

I vowed to write a letter of appreciation to Crystal for her good qualities and efforts, and immediately I was pierced by memories of when we first came together: her gentleness and compassion, my admiration of her ability to stand on her head in yoga, and how impressed I was that she wrote music. I had loved her sense of adventure when we had set off for Asia, hiking up to Annapurna Sanctuary in Nepal and then spending five weeks in India. I had seen Crystal's courage. Once we had gone with a group to Lake Tahoe for a birthday skiing trip for her. During a blizzard two of our number did not return, and twilight was falling. Crystal donned her red poncho and skied out into the landscape alone. We waited, and just as dusk fell, we saw a patch of red among the trees and watched Crystal come toward us across an open snowy valley, bringing behind her the two who had been lost. I valued so much the ways in which we had been passionate and loving with each other, all that we had shared in our first years together, and I wanted to tell her this.

That afternoon in the meditation hall Ruth directed us to sit in rows facing each other. Opening my eyes and seeing the women across from me gave me a strong sense of sangha, of being held in a community of like-minded people who were engaged in working toward the same spiritual goals. I felt grateful once again for the sisterhood of other seekers, past and present, feeling how we helped each other embody the teachings in our lives. Still, after fifteen minutes of sitting, I became lightheaded and had to lie down.

After guiding us in a meditational sweep through the body and taking the others outside for a fast walk around the meditation hall in the cold afternoon wind, Ruth told a story. She settled herself at the front of the room, arranged her voluminous skirt, peered through her glasses at us, and told of how that noontime, having lunch in her little house, she had watched a fly fall into the cream pitcher. "As quick as I could, I got her out of there!" Then Ruth had bathed the sticky fly with water. "Yes, just giving her a bath, you know, and being careful of her eyes and her antennae." Ruth lifted her chin and gave a decisive nod. "When I finished she *shook* her wings, just fluttered them a little, and then she flew away."

This simple story lodged in me. Even a fly deserves to live, I thought. Just so, my own life is precious, worth nurturing and fighting for. I needed to be convinced of this. I felt Ruth's consistency: the same concern with the many small details of life that caused her to demand loops for the kitchen rags also motivated her to take meticulous care in saving the life of a fly.

We sat in silence as the light dimmed in the meditation hall. Then the deep voice of the dinner gong entered, sent by a woman who stood halfway between meditation hall and eating hall, beating the big metal shield. When the last sound had reverberated and fallen away, Ruth's glance went from face to face in the room.

"I invite you," she said, "to eat mindfully, to remember the many labors that brought us this food, and to understand how this taking of the meal connects us with the elements that sustain all the creatures of this earth."

In the evening I had a terrifying nightmare in which Barbara, my friend and acupuncturist, drowned in a rushing river as I tried unsuccessfully to rescue her. The dream opened a deep level of pain, and after it the days at the retreat began to move in a surreal round of dreams, memories, meditation, and then lying exhausted on my back on the meditation hall floor. I had entered the hell realm, it seemed.

In Buddhism, existence is divided into six realms. In the words of Zen priest Furyu Nancy Schroeder, these realms are the stations at which the train of suffering stops. When we indulge our lusts, we inhabit the animal realm; lost in pain, believing that it will never end, we writhe in the hell realm; hungering inconsolably for what we can never have, we are hungry ghosts; when rage contorts us, we become titans bent upon destruction; and so forth. So the six realms provide a model of the human psyche.

At Dhamma Dena now I felt crushed under a huge weight. No joy awoke in me. No spaciousness opened. My senses dulled by the chemo, I could not penetrate deeply in the meditations. In my room the dream-demons tortured me.

One evening in her Dharma talk Ruth said, "When you meditate, you are opening up in deep surrender to the luminous presence of your consciousness. There you find your deeper purpose, and you can realize your motive in action." One example of this, she said, was our "taking refuge," as we did at the beginning of each retreat—taking refuge in the Buddha, the Dharma, and the Sangha. Ruth spoke forcefully: "This is an affirmation of our potential on the spiritual path. It asks us to recollect ourselves in our highest purpose: *From moment to moment, stay awake!"*

I did not feel awake, but half dead in a muddle of sensations. The next morning I dreamt that I had participated in a murder. I did not actually perform the murder, but was involved in instigating it. Every one knew what I had done, including the dead man's wife. Would they arrest me? I went on with my life in the dream, speaking in public and leading writing workshops. People told me they admired me for having the courage to continue. Somehow I knew it was necessary in order to save my life.

There were also moments of reprieve, of blessedness, during that difficult retreat. One warm afternoon sitting out behind the Samadhi House and sipping tea, I saw a baby rabbit moving in the cactus garden next to me. It streaked out into the open, poised there, its delicate ears twitching, its eyes glancing everywhere, then raced back in among the big green and white cacti. Several times it did this. A little miracle, I thought. It's *playing*—for there was neither food nor danger near.

One afternoon Ruth invited me to give my presentation on the Fourth World Conference on Women in Beijing the previous fall. I gathered my energy, and, helped by a friend, hung a sheet over the uneven plaster wall in the Samadhi House living room and positioned the slide projector. After meditation, at 3 P.M., we came over there and had "tea," a lemonade-ginger drink, with chocolate chip cookies left over from the previous night. I showed my slides and talked, connecting once again with my enthusiasm for that great convocation at the Nongovernmental Conference just outside Beijing that had brought together twenty-six thousand women from all over the world. My sister meditators watched and listened intently, and engaged me with questions. Afterward, even though I was dead tired, I felt enlivened too, for the presentation had helped me to access my effectual self, even if only for an hour.

My friend Annie Hershey, who was here at the retreat, was the one person with whom I had discussed my feelings about my radically changed body. I had asked her, carefully, timorously, how she saw me now. I think I was asking less about appearance or attractiveness, more about a deeper question: Am I still a person to you? Can you still care about me? We had had this talk in Oakland the week before, but one day at the retreat when I came back to my room I found a note from Annie on my pillow. It read:

I have been thinking about how your body has changed. To me there are new parts of you that are very beautiful, and when people ask me how you're doing, I inevitably say—no matter what you're going through—'her spirit is strong.' Your face just shines sometimes and there is a sweetness now about you. I've watched you trying to take it all in—the miscellaneous gifts and generosities of the folks who surround you—with more and more openness, delight, and deep gratitude. Which we feel from you. We couldn't do it otherwise. Yes, your hair is a little funny and you look wan, sometimes frail, but something very strong is coming through and it shows.

Most of all I want to encourage you to separate yourself from pain, and don't let yourself get caught up in dramas. You are beautiful and strong and very very alive. You are teaching all of us how to behave in such circumstances.

I love you, I'm here for you, and I admire you so much.

The immense kindness of this message entered me and opened my heart. It made me glad that people like Annie were alive in the world, and I thought of all the people in the Bay Area who were giving time and energy to help me, who supported me in such concrete ways.

Annie's energy must have buoyed me up, for that afternoon I was able to follow Ruth's guidance in the meditation hall for longer than usual, to stay alert for a whole hour. In the stillness of the desert, with the trill of a bird intruding now and then, she led us to direct our attention first to our sitting posture—to really know that we were sitting. She invited us to begin at the top of the head, sensing the bone structure of the skull and experiencing any form of aliveness that we could there. I could feel a slight tingling, a ripple of energy, under my hair.

As she guided us, I was able to explore my own head, experiencing the shape of my eyeballs resting in their sockets, tracing my nose, my tongue, my ears, the inner ear like a seashell, which controls hearing and balance. "Notice the quiet in the body as you do this," Ruth reminded us. Then she led us to encounter our tongues, to move them in our mouths, being aware of the sensations. "See that this muscle of tongue is available for your perception." She had us scrunch up our whole face, feel the strong sensation there, hold it, and then let it go, saying, "Everything is offered for the light of awareness."

Amazingly, I was able to maintain my concentration as she moved into the neck and shoulders, the chest. "Be the authentic witness," Ruth said, and I felt that my mind had gone past the witness to merge with the tissues of my arm, totally present in that aliveness. Ruth took us down the arms to the hands. "Cultivate in yourself an attitude of allowing. Notice all sensations. Notice your witnessing mind."

With meticulous slowness she directed us to experience the sensations present in our backs and chests. When we reached the hips, she asked us to make a small movement with one hip, saying this movement was "an invitation to the mind," and to feel the effect of this in our abdomens.

When we had moved down the columns of our legs, we experienced our feet. "Let the toes come to you," Ruth said softly. "Envision them. Feel their aliveness."

I realized I had stayed alert for the whole half-hour journey through my physical self. For the first time since I had arrived my body felt alive and available to me.

Leading us now in some rapid sweeps, Ruth directed, "Open to your whole body at once, where the sensations are always changing. Let the body reveal itself in its true nature. There is no solidity here: all is changing all the time. Let it change in your loving awareness."

When she rang the bell to end the session, I felt the beginning of peace in me again.

On the last evening of the retreat, after the meditation, Ruth told a story. A man with a drug habit had come to live in one of Ruth's little houses on the desert in order to escape his proximity to drugs in Los Angeles. But soon after his arrival he was diagnosed with a cancer so advanced that he was judged to be dying. He rapidly became bedridden, and it was clear that his life was ending. Ruth went to be with him as often as she could. He began the final dying process during the holiday retreat that winter, and between meditation sessions and late at night Ruth would go to sit at the man's bedside. His few friends would be there, playing music, talking, and generally agitating him. After Ruth had calmed them down, she would talk to the man, bringing him close to his body. Late one night, after giving a discourse in the meditation hall, Ruth arrived at the man's little house to find that he was in the final dying process. Guiding him with her words, she held him strongly there with his body, not letting him detour into frightening hallucinations. And she helped him let go, saying, "Give your body to the desert, give your body to the coyotes, to the baby rabbits, to the creosote bushes." As he continued to respond to her, she told him, "Give everything; don't hold any-thing back." And, "Where you are going there is so much spaciousness you can't imagine. Let yourself go there. Let yourself go." As the man died, he opened his hands and smiled.

That night, deeply released by this story, as if a tight fist of tension had relaxed, I waited at the door of the meditation hall for Ruth to come out. When she did, I asked, "If I have to die before you, will you come and help me?" She stopped, looking thoughtfully at me, and then went on walking. I didn't know how to interpret her silence, but as I lay in my bed later I kept going over the details of the story and how she had guided the man, and her advice to my living as well as my dying. Give every-thing, don't hold anything back. Give everything. I wanted that message to permeate my every moment.

The next morning when we were preparing to leave—I would be riding back with Annie in her car—Ruth, during her goodbyes to us, turned to me and said, simply, "Yes, I will."

PART FOUR

15

Listen to Your Body

Enlightenment is final defeat, not final victory.
Joko Beck

IN MY TWENTIES I made my way through the complete works of numerous writers. Married, and living in a noisy third-floor apartment in San Francisco, I would come home each night from my secretarial job, and after cooking dinner for myself and my husband and washing the dishes, I would lie on the couch in our living room and disappear for hours into those rich imagined worlds. If I felt the pull of truth in a writer's work, I would read methodically, beginning with the earliest tentative effort and moving on to the mature books, savoring the development of vision and craft, learning from the consciousness opening before me, and staying loyal even through the final, often repetitive volumes. When I had finished the last tome, my appetite would still not be satisfied, and I would read biographies of the writer. I loved the most elaborated vision, developed over a lifetime, watching it come together until it was fully textured and realized. I am loyal in the same way to my friends and mentors, whom I continue to love and appreciate no matter what configuration we may wind up in; even in the midst of discord and disappointment I find it almost impossible to give up on anyone I have truly cared for.

When I moved to my friend Nan Gefen's house, I entered a realm that brought me back to that early reading. On my first day there, after the friends who helped me move had left, I stepped out the door onto a deck made of weathered boards. Although it was summer, I had put on two jackets, a wool hat, and gloves, and I carried a blanket. Sinking down on the metal chaise longue, I lay back and covered myself from toes to chin. The hot sun pressed on my closed eyelids as I gave in to my fatigue.

I imagined that I was in the tuberculosis sanitarium described in Thomas Mann's *The Magic Mountain*.

At the International Sanatorium Berghof high in the Alps, the patients lay out on their balconies wrapped in blankets, gazing up at snow-slathered peaks. So I rested on Nan's back deck, pretending that I was one of the well-cared-for sufferers in that Bavarian haven. My body utterly devoid of energy, my condition complicated now by a badly sprained ankle, I imagined that attendants would come to help me to a hot bath, to a special meal, or healing therapies. All I had to do was lie here, the sun hot on my face, and let myself be taken care of. It was a soothing fantasy.

My move to Nan's had come as the result of several more wrenching months in Crystal's house. The resolutions I had made at Dhamma Dena melted in the cauldron of our life together as I went each week to chemotherapy and my symptoms became more acute. Our misunderstanding of one another grew ever more intense. Finally, in a therapy session, we decided that we should live separately, and since the house belonged to Crystal, it was I who would move out. Nan offered me the use of her back house for two months until a scheduled renter would move in.

My ankle, now tightly wrapped and encased in one of those big funny shoes with a thick foam sole, had been injured in a most discouraging way. I had insisted on taking a walk at Point Reyes with Sandy Butler. Coming back through perfect warm sunshine under an azure sky, on a path across meadows and flowing water, I was tired. Suddenly my foot turned and I went down, my whole weight crunching my ankle bones. Sandy half-carried me the quarter-mile to the car, and as we drove home, my ankle throbbed unbearably. It was a serious sprain, the orthopedist said, and because I was taking chemo, it would heal more slowly than usual.

Nan's back house had been designed and lived in by a well-known writer. It was a large two-story box, the downstairs a spacious study with a light wood floor and gray concrete counters, tiny state-of-the-art light fixtures suspended from a wire somewhere up near the high ceiling, a steel industrial-style refrigerator, and custom-made wooden shelves with asymmetrically curved edges. Incongruous in all that space (for the writer had taken her furniture with her when she moved out) stood a borrowed futon couch and an overstuffed chair from the Goodwill store.

In this room each morning I cooked hot cereal while listening to the tape of a chant, a long haunting invocation of Kwan Yin, the Virgin Mary, the Tibetan Buddhist goddess Tara, and the Great Goddess.

Traditional Buddhist chants serve different purposes in the several traditions: to remind us of moral and ethical principles, to express "taking refuge" in the Buddha, Dharma, and Sangha, to pay homage to certain deities or qualities, and to connect outer and inner realities, arousing transformative vibrations in the body; they promote concentration, and help to focus the mind on some quality to be developed or to make a vow to accomplish something.

But the chant with which I began each day had been created by a singer-songwriter friend of mine, expressing her own connection with the bodhisattva Kwan Yin while honoring her original Catholic background and her veneration of the Great Goddess. Built upon the repeated phrase "She who hears the cries of the world" above layered drums and other instruments, this twenty-minute chant with its blended voices wove a supportive fabric of sound around me as I teetered on my ankle-cast, stirring at the stove and swallowing my nausea at the smell of cooked grains. The pulse of this song helped prepare me for each day.

Upstairs in the cathedral-like bedroom, I had spread a cloth on the floor in the corner and propped up the photographs of my brother, Maurine Stuart, Lex Hixon, and my parents. I replicated the altar from the living room at Crystal's house and placed my meditation cushion before it. But when I tried to sit in meditation, I drooped with fatigue, as I had at Dhamma Dena.

So with Ruth Denison as my inspiration, I went to the simplest practice. Just as she had done with the broom, telling herself, "I take the broom. I am sweeping," I set myself to be fully aware of each activity. Soon I realized that this attention was necessary not only for my state of mind, but for my safety and whatever comfort I might manage.

In the stark white bathroom each morning, I met the challenge of brushing my teeth. My mouth tasted of chemicals, and whenever I smelled the toothpaste, nausea rose in my throat. It took all my concentration to brush and swallow while suppressing the urge to vomit.

Gazing at my sore, dry, reddened eyes in the mirror, I opened a drawer to take out special eye drops, thick and viscous, that adhered to the surface of the lids. Gratefully I felt the cool liquid ease my eyes, though I knew that the itching would return within an hour.

Then came the journey down the stairway. My injured ankle had thrown off my sense of balance, so that I felt my fragility and the potential danger in the polished wood steps. "I am going down one step," I told myself. "I feel the wood under my foot. I let my weight down on this foot. Now I'm moving the cane to the next step down. Balance. Bring weight onto the foot. Now center myself to get ready for the next step."

In this manner I made my way down to the little kitchenette, where I swallowed the many supplements, vitamins, and Chinese herbs that supported my immune system to tolerate the chemotherapy. Then I cooked the oatmeal and made a cup of tea, saying to myself "Now I place the sauce pan on the burner. Now I stir the cereal." Accompanying me in these preparations were the recorded voices intoning the chant.

I hobbled across the floor to the big worn chair, placed my breakfast on an end-table, sat down, and raised my injured ankle to rest on a straight chair. Taking a deep breath, I gazed around me. The walls, a pale yellow, looked lemony in the morning light; through the windows I saw the trees and flowers of the garden, where goldfish swam in a small pond. There were no freeway noises here. I heard only the songs of birds.

Slowly I ate the cereal, chewing and swallowing past the incipient nausea. ("Lifting spoon, putting cereal in mouth." I told myself what I was doing. "Putting down the spoon. Chewing.") I experienced the sensations of mouth and tongue and throat. I felt my hand lift the spoon again, staying close to this mind-body process that was myself.

When the bowl was empty and the chant had fallen away into silence, I rewarded myself for the good work done. I picked up the book from the end table and began to read Rumer Godden. Godden is a British novelist who grew up in colonial India; born in 1907, she must be a very old lady now if she is still alive. Her best-known book, *Black Narcissus*, details the disorientation and breakdown of five Catholic nuns in a castle-like convent in the Himalayas. In 1946 it was made into a movie starring Deborah Kerr: a brooding, visually stunning film. I had found Rumer Godden through *In This House of Brede*, a novel about the prioress of a Catholic nunnery in England. I had always been drawn to and fascinated by the monastic vocation. Some years before, I had journeyed to Sri Lanka to spend six weeks living as a Buddhist nun. (In Theravada Buddhism, one can take robes for short periods of time.) There on a tiny island in a lake, at the nunnery established by Ayya Khema, the German-born nun who was a leader in the movement to achieve better conditions for Buddhist female monastics, I lived the life of contemplation and inwardness. Cloistered on that tropical, jungly island, I was able to go deeply into my practice, and to experience the shared life of renunciants who lived, meditated, and studied together.

While the subject-matter of Godden's books interested me, I was also intrigued by the author's psychology, for Godden lived in two psychic worlds, always dealing with the tension between the richly exotic India of her girlhood and the proper England of her later years. Now in my hibernation—hidden away in the back of a house—I sought out her resonant prose. Whenever someone drove me to my chemo appointment, I would ask to stop at a library, and look for yet another Godden book. I needed to see how differently people met life and confronted death. Godden gave flesh to the numerous philosophies of the East, exploring them through the characters of gardeners, cooks, and public servants, and through the life of the land and the great sacred Ganges river itself.

Almost every morning as I sat reading, I would hear the door between this back house and Nan's house open, and Nan would appear. With her perceptive blue eyes, she would regard me across the expanse of floor. "How're you doing?" she would ask, and after I answered, she would announce, "I'm going to the store today—what can I get you? Yogurt? Peaches? Can I tempt you with ice cream?" Then, at almost every visit, before she went back through the door, she would say, "I'm so very glad you're here."

When she left I would sit with my head lowered. To be told that I was welcome, that I was cherished, touched me in a tender place. Nan's statement each time she made it was a gift to me.

During the long July days, after my morning ritual, I would do some work at the wooden table near the door. Then, moving awkwardly on my sprained ankle, I would go to the polished concrete counter and put fruit and yogurt in a blender to make a smoothie, one of the few substances I could get down my throat. Then I would climb the stairs, crawl into bed, and go to sleep again. Afternoon would be filled with an errand (I could still drive). I came home to sleep again. At dinnertime I would receive the visit of a woman (a different friend each day) bringing soup, perhaps a white carton of wonton soup from a Chinese restaurant or something she had made herself. While she sat watching me, I would do my best to eat it. Then after another nap, if I were teaching a class in my house that evening, I would sweep the floor ("Now I am holding the broom, now I am sweeping") and steel myself to be usefully present for two hours.

Finally the time would come to lie down in the great expanse of the king-size bed in the upstairs room, to stare exhausted at a borrowed TV, watching the superbly-toned bodies of Olympic athletes performing feats so far from my physical reality that they might as well have been taking place on the moon.

So the days passed. I became more bony and gray-tinged. The skin on my fingers cracked and bled. My eyes hurt all the time. And a day came when I vomited the wonton soup, and knew I would no longer be able to tolerate it. Bill and Sally began to worry about me when they discovered that I had lost forty pounds.

My sixtieth birthday was approaching. At the beginning of the year I had made plans to have a birthday celebration with all of my friends, as I had done on my fiftieth birthday. But I had had to give up the plan several months ago—only one more of the losses the cancer and treatment had wrought. Now I had no plans at all for my birthday and no energy to make any. I experienced my life force as a flame inside my chest; a pilot light that had diminished month by month before the onslaught of the chemo until it burned now only as a tiny wavering flame, sending almost no heat out to my body. The light grew smaller and flickered more weakly every day. I retreated into myself, living internally, in order to tend it and try my hardest to keep it burning.

One night I lay awake in the big bed, disturbed by what my life had become. That day I had gone to see Barbara for acupuncture. Barbara had felt my pulses, looked at my tongue, and inserted the needles. But when it was time for me to leave, she put a steadying hand on my arm. "Sandy," she said, "I think you have maxed out on the chemo. Your body can't take any more." She let that sink in, and then said, "I will support you in quitting the treatments if that's what you decide to do."

I sat up in bed, turned on the light, propped some pillows behind me and leaned back. The light threw a buttery circle out over the wood floor, touching the elegant white stove on its concrete platform, my meditation cushion before my makeshift altar. The house was silent except for its occasional strange nighttime cracking noises. The blackness of the sky pressed against the windows, as still as a held breath.

Rubbing at my burning eyes, I wondered, "How will I earn a living if I can't read or write?" When my hand rested again on the comforter, I saw the bones of my wrist, my watch hanging loosely there. I now weighed less than I had as a skinny twenty-year-old. Being so thin made me feel completely at the mercy of the outside world. "If I can't eat," I asked myself, "how will I survive?" That night when I had brushed my teeth, I had vomited up the smoothie I had had for dinner. "This is unacceptable!" I thought. "I have to get my body back!" But I did not know how to do that.

My sixtieth birthday brought yet another physical challenge. The Wandering Menstruals, Crystal, and my writing class had each celebrated this juncture with me in the week preceding, but on the actual day I sat alone in my Goodwill chair, reading Rumer Godden with greatly flawed concentration.

A friend visiting from Massachusetts came to see me. Ellen, writer, computer expert, and psychic, arrived with her characteristic breeziness to take me shopping. She had given me her old computer (which for me was very new) and now she was taking me to buy a printer. I put on my several coats and knitted hat, strapped on my foam-rubber cast, and hobbled out to Ellen's little red rental car.

As we made our way across town and down Ashby Avenue, I enjoyed Ellen's witty account of life in western Massachusetts, where she had been living for only a short time. But as we sat waiting for a red light to change, suddenly Ellen looked up at the rearview mirror. "Uh-oh!" she exclaimed. I leaned forward, turning my head to look back. At that instant a huge blue van crashed into us, making a loud crunching sound. Our little car lurched forward, and my neck jerked, my body tightening against the impact.

Half an hour later we were riding in a tow truck, the red car with its mashed-in trunk dragging behind us, out to the Oakland airport where Ellen had rented it. Several hours later we arrived, in a different car, at the office of a chiropractor friend, who examined me and told me I had very serious whiplash. My neck felt locked in place.

When finally I got back to my bedroom, I sank gratefully into the bed, and lay considering. Now besides a sprained ankle, I had a damaged neck. What was the message of this latest disaster? For the first time since being told that I had cancer I was frightened, for it seemed that the chemo had brought me to such a state of weakness that I had no resilience. The flame burned lower each day. Was I dying? The material world had begun to batter me, damaging my body even further. Could I possibly stop the chemo treatments? Dr. Cutting, head of Oncology, had emphasized that one must undergo forty-eight weeks of continuous treatment. I had done only twenty-five weekly treatments, and that already seemed like a huge number to me! Given my high sensitivity to drugs, couldn't I assume that the chemo had done its job already and could be stopped? But no one had offered any modifying options in following the protocol: if you accepted the treatment, you did it for forty-eight weeks—end of story. I knew how adamant the doctors were and how they minimized the "side effects." Worst of all, who could know whether there had actually been any errant cancer cells in my system? And if there had been, who could know whether the chemo had eradicated them? Perhaps they were already lodged in my liver. Or maybe there hadn't been any in the first place. It was enormously frustrating to me that the treatment was based on statistics and speculation rather than concrete evidence.

So I agonized. As long as my course had been mapped out for me, as long as I had known what to do each day, I had been able to live each moment with some equanimity. Now I was caught, both afraid to continue the chemo and afraid to stop taking it.

That night, despite my deep fatigue, I slept only a few hours.

In the morning, ensconced in my chair in the living room, my book unopened next to me, I remembered the last thing Barbara had said to me as I left her acupuncture office: "Listen to your body." I sat looking out the windows at the trees bright in the summer sunshine. "Listen to your body." Maybe the answer lay there, rather than in my wildly speculating mind. After all, it was my body that was receiving the chemicals, enduring the cellular changes and most of the diminishment. It made sense to consult this physical entity and take in its experience. I would gather my energies in order to meditate.

I sat up a little straighter and, closing my eyes, directed my attention inward, taking note of my sitting body, its weight on the chair. I visited the ache in my ankle and the tightness of my neck. Then I began to pay attention to my breath, letting it connect me strongly, bringing all my meager forces to bear. I followed my breath down into my chest, visiting lungs and heart. I explored my belly, site of the surgery, the cavern filled with the many feet of coiled intestine, the dark blot of my liver.

For a long time I stayed there, my breath like a thread sewing mind and body together. I followed it in and out, in and out, and rested with utter receptivity in the recesses of my body until the answer came: "This is too much poison for me. The chemicals have done their job and now they're killing me."

The message was perfectly clear. I sat still, allowing myself to fully receive it, and I knew what I must decide.

The decision brought with it a new challenge. I would have to confront Dr. Cutting, a man who did not take kindly to insubordination. I anticipated that he would try to bully me into obedience, scare me with statistics, berate and intimidate me to make me continue the treatments. So I prepared carefully. I wrote out all my reasons for quitting chemotherapy. And I asked Sandy Butler to go with me to my next appointment, since she was experienced in talking to doctors.

The Oncology Clinic was particularly busy that day, with every chair filled. Bill and Sally went about their duties with their usual warmth and efficiency. Gondica came out to greet me. And as usual, we waited. In the car driving here, Sandy and I had gone over my written-out reasons for quitting—the litany of weakness, weight loss, nausea, cracking skin, and sore eyes—and she promised to speak up for me if Dr. Cutting pushed me to continue. Now we sat side by side on the plastic chairs, and soon gave up on conversing. I felt myself resort to an attitude I had adopted as a child when standing up to my father. Now and then, in the face of his authority, I had known I could not obey him. I went to a place in myself that was unyielding, which I vowed I would not abandon, no matter what. This had happened only a few times in my childhood, but every instance was indelible, for each time the danger had been palpable. I had watched my brother defy my father and be beaten down, sometimes physically. I knew I had to risk that; I had to be ready, even if he hit me, to stand my ground. On the other hand I knew how much he loved me. He had only ever spanked me once, and then never touched me in anger again. I was not my brother. So I had said, "No, I won't." My father had become very still, looking down at me from his great height, his big carpenter's hands open at his sides. He looked amazed, then puzzled. Then he retreated behind an expression I could not read, and without a word he turned his back and left the room.

How lucky I had been that my father had not bent me to his will.

Because he had not, I knew I could oppose Dr. Cutting, here where my very life was at stake. I felt how fortunate I was in other ways too—to have access to alternative healers like Barbara, and most of all to the meditation practice of attending to this body-mind process, which could bring me close enough to hear what my physical self experienced.

My name was called, and Sandy and I were ushered into a curtained cubicle to wait for Dr. Cutting. I sat on a chair, clutching my notes, and Sandy leaned against a wall. "Hey, girl," she said, "it's going to be fine." I wasn't so sure.

Cutting entered. A short man, unassuming and blunt, without the air of special importance that surrounds many doctors, he was attired in a rumpled shirt and casual jacket rather than a starched white coat. A doctor of long experience with cancer, he was the top man in Oncology, much appreciated by the medical staff, who found him to be an excellent teacher and practitioner, and disliked by many others because of his authoritarian, impatient manner.

"So how're you doing?" he asked as he hurried into our enclosure and picked up my hefty hospital chart.

"Not good," I replied.

"Hmm?" He was peering down at my folder, flipping through the pages.

Not daring to look at Sandy, I began, "Dr. Cutting, I'm going to have to quit the chemotherapy."

He stopped turning pages, closed the file, and laid it on the desk. His eyes behind his glasses widened in surprise as he leaned back against the counter and folded his arms over his chest.

The gesture was not reassuring. Looking at my notes, I rushed ahead, describing my symptoms in as vivid detail as possible, giving him my rationale for stopping, point by point. When I fell silent, Dr. Cutting stood thinking for a moment.

Then he said, "Well, if this is all you can take, stop."

I stared at him.

Dr. Cutting began to pace the few feet of cubicle space, and he talked to Sandy and me. "As doctors, our knowledge is limited. We hit upon the forty-eight-week protocol arbitrarily. No one really knows whether a shorter course of treatment would work as well. In order to find that out, we'd have to do studies, and frankly there isn't the kind of money for studies on colon cancer that there is, for instance, for breast cancer. When they first started giving chemo for certain kinds of breast cancer, they did it for a year. Then they did studies that indicated six months was enough, then more studies that led them to shorten the course of therapy further, and so on. But with colon cancer we don't have the study results to warrant that."

He stopped pacing and gestured at my chart. "Also, we're aware that every patient is an individual case, with a different tolerance of the drugs and sensitivity to them. So you see we're working in the dark, in a way, with very crude and partial information."

He lifted his shoulders in a shrug while Sandy and I gazed at him, speechless.

Then Dr. Cutting shifted into high gear again, leaning down to open my file and scribble in it, talking all the while.

"So what we'll do is this. You'll come in for a colonoscopy in October—that's just a year from your surgery—and if that's clear, then you'll come in every six months for blood tests and a checkup, and you'll have a colonoscopy the following year. I'll have Sally make you an appointment for October in the G.I. lab."

He had finished writing in the file, closed it, and was halfway out the door. I stood up.

"So that's it," Dr. Cutting said. We watched him turn on his heel and walk away from us down the row of cubicles.

Sandy and I stared at each other. Apparently, my determination to follow my own perceptions and intuition had given Dr. Cutting permission to drop his usual manner and talk to me not like a patient but like another intelligent human being. This transformation in itself, as well as the information he had given me, felt like support for my decision.

Leaving the hospital that day, coming out into the mild July afternoon, I realized what had happened. The chemo ordeal had officially ended.

PART FIVE

16

Ordinary Wisdom

*We are fundamentally alone, and there is nothing anywhere to
hold on to. Moreover, this is not a problem. In fact, it allows us
to finally discover a completely unfabricated state of being.*

Pema Chodron

OUR CANCER SUPPORT GROUP was saddened by the death of Joyce. She
had realized that her years'-long battle with cancer was over, had signed
up for hospice care, and surrendered to the dying process. Rick Fields
went to visit her at home, where her husband cared for her, and brought
us accounts of how she was as she drifted in and out of consciousness. We
sat in our circle in the basement room, and I felt both sorrow and relief,
for I had been witness to Joyce's suffering as she submitted to each new
treatment and struggled to live. I was sorry that she had to die, and yet
her death would bring her release from that suffering.

While Joyce entered her dying process, I began the return to health,
and her example let me know how lucky I was. Slowly I made my way
out of the dense chemo-fog that for twenty-five weeks had obscured the
contours of my previous life, allowing me such limited vision, activity, and
expectations. Any idea that in a week or a month I would have recovered
from its effects soon had to be abandoned; but gradually, day by day,
month by month, the fog thinned in spots, and things that were formerly obscured, appeared again—I regained some capacities, and my discomfort lessened. My decision had marked the end of my focus on
disease and inaugurated a time of healing: looking ahead, I imagined
being able to eat, to take a walk, to read without discomfort.

But the first big project was to move again. I would be living with a
friend in a second-floor apartment not far from Crystal's house. I found

it comforting that I would be staying in a familiar neighborhood. Jeannie, my future roommate, had been a public figure in the seventies, involved in an intensely politicized child custody case that was the first to publicly challenge the court's removal of children from gay and lesbian parents. Her sons were grown now, and she lived for the most part in the country in Northern California, but she kept an apartment in Oakland. She had explained to me that she would mostly be absent during the autumn, and I would have the apartment to myself.

I kept up my *Magic Mountain* regime at Nan's house, lying on the deck in the sun whenever possible. After breakfast I read Rumer and Jon Godden's *Two Under the Indian Sun*, a memoir of their childhood in India. I fantasized a trip down the Ganges. Crystal and I, in our five weeks in India, had gone out on the great river in Benares, the holy city, and had seen the smoke of a cremation on the wide steps of the burning ghat. I imagined long days on a ship floating down the whole length of the Ganges, observing the activity of its busy shores, which Rumer and Jon brought vividly to life. Illness allows for a certain freedom: becalmed by disease, one can indulge any fantasy.

More mundane, closer-to-home events encouraged me. One day, leaving the chiropractor's office, where I went for regular treatments for my whiplash, I bought a burrito and sat at a little table on the sidewalk. Carefully I took the first bite and chewed. Beans and rice and salsa—it actually tasted good!

Again my "sangha" gathered to help me move the ten blocks to Jeannie's apartment. Three of the Wandering Menstruals called upon their nearly grown sons to carry out boxes to a borrowed truck. In the kitchen two of my helpers who had met for the first time while hefting my desk found a strong connection. Terry, a psychiatrist and prison activist, began talking animatedly to Roxanne, a friend from the Graduate Theological Union, about state psychiatric care for mentally ill inmates. Soon they were deep into reminiscences of the Kudzu alliance in the Carolinas, a coalition of anti-nuclear groups that worked to halt construction of nuclear plants and push for disarmament. Therapists and social workers, artists and lawyers, college students and a professor, mothers, sons, and fathers—mine was a lively, good-humored crew, everyone telling everyone else what to do.

They wrestled my belongings up the narrow steps to Jeannie's apartment to the two small rooms that were to be mine, while I wandered about giving directions when asked, feeling inadequate and exceedingly grateful. I was amazed at Lenore Friedman, author of *Meetings with Remarkable Women*, a book about Buddhist women teachers. Sixty-seven years old at the time, small and delicate-looking, she lifted huge boxes and plodded springily up the stairs with them, as if this were something she did every day. Nancy Schmit, one of my writing students, volunteered her van and organized the packing with formidable efficiency.

Crystal was absent from the house, but had left many notes to instruct us on everything that was to be done. With our counselor, she and I had made lists of which objects were hers, and which mine; her notes reminded me not only of our decisions but the arguments that had preceded them.

Moving day was long, hugely exhausting, and tolerably entertaining as my helpers made jokes and teased each other.

That night I came home to Nan's house and got in bed. It was a Sunday. I lay in the huge bed in the high-ceilinged room, and the mud of nostalgia began to gather and suck me down. Sunday had been my and Crystal's special day to be together, when we would set out for Point Reyes or some other outdoor destination, and hike or bicycle for hours, enjoying the trees, the ocean, the exertion of our healthy bodies. On the long drive back to Oakland, in the twilight or the dark, our talk would meander gently from our work to Crystal's daughter's doings up in Washington, from the state of the world to a future trip to Africa and how we might start planning for it. At home we would get into bed and watch a movie, and then go happily to sleep. Now, lying alone in the bed at Nan's, I longed for that easy intimacy, that reliable routine of pleasure and satisfaction with someone I knew so well.

It was the beginning of loneliness, obscured during the time at Nan's by the necessity to put my longings and griefs aside. I had needed to reside strongly in the moment, to stay loyal to the demands of my struggling, depleted body, simply to do the next thing that might help me live through the ordeal. Now the storm had quieted, and I felt washed up on the beach, like a piece of seaweed torn from its mooring.

I rolled over to the side of the big bed and got out. In the stark white bathroom I turned on the light and stood looking in the mirror, searching the face that stared back at me.

I had always had a moon-face, round with firm cheeks. The cheeks I saw in the mirror now sagged against the bone. A network of tiny meshed lines had appeared on my skin from my lower eyelids down across my cheeks. I remembered my mother's face, with its high cheekbones and thin lips, her pale redhead's skin fine and smooth until she died. People had always judged her to be much younger than she was, and I had shared that youthful appearance, before the chemo. Now I looked ancient, my face carved in grooves and hollows, my green eyes peering warily out at the world. Still, after two weeks without chemo, my skin had begun to look more pink and less gray.

I heard Nan's voice speaking to me from our dinner together several days before: "you look very young and very old, both at the same time— like a preadolescent girl, new and eager," she tilted her head to the side, regarding me, adding, "or...I guess I'd say, ready."

Looking at myself in the mirror, I saw the skin of my skull peeking through the thin whorls of gray hair, which I had cut very short when it began to fall out, and I heard another voice. Roxanne, visiting me in the hospital months ago, studying me as I sat up in bed in a patterned gown, had said, "You look like a Dr. Seuss character." I had flinched, seeing a tall ungainly creature with long wobbly neck topped by a small round head. Did I really appear so ridiculous? Roxanne stood grinning at me with such delight that I let myself go past my initial hurt feelings to see that I probably did look like a silly Dr. Seuss character. Roxanne added, "That's how I know you're really okay."

I turned out the light in the snowy bathroom and made my way back to the huge raft of my bed. My face in the mirror had told me nothing I didn't already know. It was simply a map of the territory I had crossed. I surrendered to the bed and the darkness, faceless again, my body opened to the mattress's support and my mind softening within minutes into sleep.

The next day I left my sanctuary at Nan's house and officially moved to the two small rooms in Jeannie's apartment where I was to live. The apartment was spacious, with many windows and a back deck; the rooms were decorated lovingly by Jeannie, who was an accomplished sculptor, with many touches from Italy, where she had lived for some years. To accommodate me, Jeannie had moved into the large living-dining area, which closed off to make a small two-room suite; we shared the kitchen and bathroom. My two rooms were at opposite sides of the kitchen, so that to go from study to bedroom I had to make my way past the kitchen table. But for the moment, the arrangement seemed fine to me, particularly since I was still so ill that I mostly wanted a place to put my bed so that I could crawl into it.

Though I did not know Jeannie well, I had always respected her, and in the infrequent conversations we had had about art I was impressed with a certain very subtle intelligence she expressed. She was still politically concerned and vocal, and she regularly did yoga and meditated, both at home and at the Siddha Yoga ashram in Oakland. I myself went to the ashram each Friday morning to eat breakfast and drink their excellent chai. So Jeannie was in some sense a known quantity, in other ways a mystery.

Our building stood on a busy corner near the main thoroughfare of MacArthur Boulevard. Through the windows in our second-floor rooms, we heard the loud talking of passersby, the roar of hotrodders. Often, in the middle of the night, I would be awakened by the buzz of skateboarders rolling past through the empty streets. In the house next door, just under my bedroom window, twin toddlers screamed sometimes for as long as fifteen minutes at a time, a behavior I never understood, although I was fairly sure they were not being abused. It seemed that they egged each other on, and were not stopped by the parents or babysitters. Outside on the pavement, drug deals occasionally went down, the man across the street had been mugged in his garage, and car windows were now and then smashed to allow the car to be rifled. At times our apartment throbbed under a barrage of sound.

Some of this I did not yet know on that first day I moved in. It was 8:30 P.M. I had eaten part of a can of lentil soup. Now I sat in the tiny room that was to be my study. All my files, notes, manuscripts, letters, and records had been gathered into the cardboard cartons stacked around me. My friends had filled the boxes; I had little idea of which cartons held what. I leaned my elbows on my knees, and gazed at the floor. It was as if I had landed here in a little bubble, outside the flow of normal life. As the fog slowly drifted from my mental landscape, I was beginning to see my true situation. At Nan's house, even though I knew that Crystal and I had agreed to live separately, I was too ill to really think about it. Now, sitting in the noisy little room among the jumble of my things, I remembered moving into the house with Crystal three years before, my delight as I discovered the storage space in my study, which we had converted from a dining room. In the gracious living room, with its high ceiling, comfortable furniture, and beautiful large potted plants, I had spent many hours reading, had taught many classes. The kitchen with its blond-stained cabinets, the little breakfast nook where we had eaten and talked, the bedroom and backyard...I had loved the house that Crystal and I shared. In so many ways, our life together had supported and nourished me. Now I understood, Oh, I no longer live there. It's not my home anymore.

This tiny, cluttered room seemed very bleak, particularly as I began to hear loud rock music through the wall from the neighboring apartment. Anger simmered in me, and I turned it on myself: I had screwed up my relationship so badly that my partner could not be with me emotionally in the hardest times! I let the rage go on for a while, recognizing both its futility and its inevitability. Ayya Khema, addressing the issue of anger in Buddhism, had said, "Because we are human beings, we experience anger and greed as well as all the other emotions. So when you feel anger, there is no need to judge yourself or try to suppress it. But it would be wrong to vent your ill-will on another person. Better to simply observe it until it loses momentum and falls away, so you see once again the impermanence of everything." I knew I had often failed in this, that while I was able to be patient with students and friends, I had sometimes acted out my anger on Crystal with impatience and sarcasm. Looking back, I found a lot to regret.

Looking forward, I saw nothing certain, for I did not know whether Jeannie and I would get along when she came back here to live. And a larger question loomed: until I underwent the colonoscopy in October, I could not be certain that I was free of cancer.

I sat astonished, looking at what remained of my life.

Still, that night as I lay in bed, assaulted by the street noises, I was grateful, knowing how lucky I was to have a warm bed in a safe room. While it seemed everything else had left me, yet I had this. Sandy Butler had lent me a long goose-down-filled coat, and I had spread it over the blankets to make my bed even warmer. I knew that people as sick as I was were huddled on cold concrete, propped in doorways: in my mind arose the face of a young woman covered with red sores, probably the marks of advanced AIDS—I had seen her sitting cross-legged on the sidewalk late at night in San Francisco, her two small children, dull-eyed, leaning against her, as she lifted her hand to beg for money to pay for a room.

I knew how fortunate I was to be here in this bed under my piled blankets as I pulled Sandy's down coat up under my chin, coveting the bed's warmth and softness.

The next morning, I drove to North Berkeley to clean where I had been living in Nan's back house. After sweeping the floors and scrubbing the kitchen and bathroom, I came upon a book on the floor behind the couch. It was my well-thumbed copy of Pema Chodron's lectures. I had met Pema ten years before, when she had spoken at a Women and Buddhism conference at Vajradhatu in Boulder. Just my age, with a cheery round face and shaven head, swathed in the maroon robes of a Tibetan Buddhist nun, Pema had spoken hesitantly and modestly. I had liked her a lot. I interviewed her for *Turning the Wheel*, learning that she had been a rather bohemian mother of two before taking the robes, a past that endeared her to me. Over the years since then Pema had developed into a powerful teacher, but she remained unassuming—a perfectly ordinary-seeming woman whose words and example have become profoundly inspiring to many, reaching beyond the Buddhist community to touch a wide range of people.

Tired from cleaning, I slumped on the couch and opened Pema's book. Reading, I heard her voice, talking about the patience that is necessary for healing. Slow down, she advised. Don't be in a hurry. We have plenty of time to let things evolve at their own speed. To heal, she suggested, we need to develop less resistance to what is going on, learn to trust that there is "ordinary wisdom" available in every moment—and that it may be even more available in the hard and painful moments.

I once heard Pema describing a film about Mother Theresa's work in Calcutta. It happened to be a movie I had seen. Immediately, the scene unfolded in my mind: A deformed child, with a big head and twisted limbs, thrashed in a bed, twisting and writhing, his eyes dark with terror. A nun came close, leaned over the bed, and began to rub the child's chest and belly, simply stroking him. At first the little boy kept thrashing just as frantically, then, his face attentive as if listening, he seemed to feel the comforting hand; gradually he calmed, his actions slowing, until finally he lay still. He gazed up at the nun, his great black eyes shining with gratitude. Pema asked us to imagine that each of us is, at once, the frantic, suffering child and the comforting woman.

Looking at the ceiling, I pondered the story. Could I possibly develop the compassion and the patience to accept my real, imperfect, suffering self? Could I simply allow my suffering to *be here,* not judge it, and not struggle to escape it? For an instant I saw, as if through a tiny window briefly opened, how differently these moments would feel to me if I could let them simply be my life. Why are we so often convinced that we're in the wrong story? Oh no, *this* isn't what's supposed to happen! Surely I wasn't *supposed* to lose my home, my relationship, and my health! As I squirmed internally, I also began to smile, because I could imagine Pema watching me. I heard her voice, amused and infinitely kind, as it most often is. "Hang in there," she said. "Try to lighten up and be patient with yourself."

I drove back to Jeannie's apartment, climbed up the stairs, and collapsed into bed, promising myself to open more boxes when I awoke.

These several months were a complicated time, with moments of joy winding through the difficulties like sweet rivers of grace. While my study was still mostly contained in boxes, I received the copy-edited manuscript of *Opening the Lotus* from my publisher and began the grueling work of checking the corrections, making final changes, and inputting both the copyeditor's and my own alterations onto a computer file. During the ten days of this painstaking labor my printer refused to obey the computer; I found myself driving back and forth to the repairman, struggling with impatience.

There were small epiphanies. One day at the grocery store I bought a bottle of ranch dressing, just to try. At home I tasted it, and my world lit up. Somehow this combination of sweet and sour—buttermilk, egg yolks, garlic, and vinegar—cut through the deadness of my damaged tissues and spoke directly to my taste buds. Not only could I taste it, but it sparkled in my mouth. I had not been able to eat salad for months. Now I bought lettuce and fresh spinach, red onion, broccoli, cauliflower, tomatoes, and mushrooms. I concocted the salad, poured ranch dressing over the top, and took it out on the deck to eat. A stunningly happy experience, as the dressing called up the flavors of the vegetables. I munched, gazing out over the rooftops of Oakland, enjoying the sun on my arms, realizing what was happening here: I was eating salad!

Crystal and I continued to meet with the counselor in grim sessions focused most often on questions of money. During the inevitable wrangling, I would find myself wracked with annoyance. I did my best to do the *tonglen* practice, breathing in distrust and rage, and breathing out a sense of relaxation and well-being. The practice helped, at times, to soften me to Crystal's perspective, to prevent me from answering back too quickly. Occupied with the effort of breathing, of imagining the dark cloud of hostility entering me and being transformed, and then with each outbreath summoning up the energies of kindness and patience, I had to be silent, to hold on and wait to see whether I could be clear about what was going on. Sometimes the *tonglen* would actually bring me to a calmer, more spacious attitude. At other times nothing could stem the flood of my huge irritation at Crystal's demands.

Driving home from one of those sessions, I stopped at the gym where I used to exercise. With a guest pass I went in to swim for the first time since my surgery. The covered pool-room had glass windows at the peak of the roof, through which sunlight fell to illuminate the blue bottom of the pool. I lowered myself into the water, thrilling to its touch as it enfolded me. I swam slowly, stretching my thin arms out before me, looking through my goggles down at the sun-warmed bottom, where reflected ripples formed, undulated, and broke apart—back and forth, back and forth I swam, suspended, having entered a realm softer than that of air. And I was filled with immense happiness.

In Jeannie's living room I began to teach an evening class called Major Transitions. The eight women who signed up were all experiencing significant changes in their lives, and most of these junctures were problematical. Each week I led the group in exercises to examine our patterns in reacting to change, and encouraged the women to deal creatively with this opportunity through writing and art. The class, set up for others, was a patent attempt to confront my own losses. While I kept the students' needs in the forefront, the group made a partial container for my own grief.

In my bedroom I had arranged my altar against the baseboard under the windows; it was wedged between the bookcase and the stand for the TV set. My bed nearly filled the room, leaving just enough space to sit on my pillow before the candles and incense holder. This altar was simpler than the previous ones, with a photograph of the famous statue of Kwan Yin in Kansas City and only a few of the images of my dead ones.

Sitting before it each morning, I picked up the thick volume of the *Majjima Nikaya*, or the *Middle Length Discourses* of the Buddha. Every day I read one of these *suttas* and the attendant copious notes, doing my best to enter the Buddha's world of 2,500 years ago and experience the way his message was presented and taught then. One morning I re-read the twelfth sutta, the Mahasihanada Sutta, the "Greater Discourse on the Lion's Roar," which is the Buddha's assertion of his own spiritual mastery. The words were stirring. Responding to a challenge to his spiritual authority, the Buddha declares himself to be "…all-enlightened, walking by knowledge, blessed, knowing all worlds, the matchless tamer of the human heart, teacher of gods and men, the Lord of enlightenment." He enumerates his yogic powers: "to pass in and out of the solid earth as if it were water, to walk on the water's unbroken surface as if it were the solid earth, to glide in state through the air like a bird on the wing, to touch and to handle the moon and sun in their power and might…" and speaking of himself in the third person, asserts, "He is the Lord who, with the Ear Celestial…hears both heavenly and human sounds…. He is the Lord who with his own heart comprehends the heart of other creatures and of other men so as to know them for just what they are…" I heard the words almost as if they were spoken in the room, and I began to imagine a conversation between the Buddha and Patacara, one of his enlightened female contemporaries.

Patacara had been a teacher, with a large following of women students. She had suffered great tragedy, losing her husband to snakebite, her children to flood and the attacks of animals, and her parents and siblings to a storm, all in the space of one day. Driven to madness, she had wandered the streets dressed in rags, babbling her sorrow, until one day the Buddha had encountered her and through his own mind-power had brought her back to sanity. When she told him why she grieved, the Buddha told her that he could not help her. He explained to her that just as she was now shedding tears for her dead children and relatives, in her numberless previous lives she had shed similar tears over similar losses, more than enough to fill "the waters of the four oceans." Hearing the Buddha's words, seeing the path of no salvation, Patacara's grief became lighter. When the Buddha saw this he told her that no parent, husband, or child could protect her from suffering and death. He advised her, given this, to purify her own conduct and set out on the path to *nibbana*, or liberation. Just by hearing him, Patacara was set upon the path, and she asked to be ordained. The Buddha took her to the *bhikkhunis* (nuns), and let her be admitted to the renunciants order. Not long after, doing her practice, Patacara achieved the highest level of realization, becoming an *arahat* (enlightened one). Soon women came to seek help from her, five hundred of them it was said, most often mothers whose children had died; and Patacara taught them the truth of no consolation, helping them liberate themselves from their paralysis of grief, and led them to practice the Dharma and plant the seeds of their own freedom.

I imagined an encounter between the aged Buddha and the equally old Patacara, both by that time seasoned spiritual teachers and leaders near the end of their lives. In the Mahasihanada Sutta it is explicit that the Buddha is eighty years old; Patacara might be roughly the same age, or even slightly older. I visualized two aged, dark-skinned people, dressed in brown robes, seated in the forest, talking together about their lives.

They would roar their lions' roars. But Patacara's roar would be critically different from the Buddha's. The Buddha character spoke the text of the *sutta*, graphically describing the many austerities that he had imposed upon himself before deciding to adopt the middle path. ("After this wise, in divers fashions, have I lived to torment and to torture my body;—to such a length in asceticism have I gone.") Then Patacara could tell her story, and we would see that the Buddha's austerities were chosen by himself, while the tragedy that drove Patacara mad was imposed upon her. He had freely opted to confront the suffering of life. She had had no choice but to do so, and this no doubt says something about the difference between the lives of men and women in ancient India. In order to "go forth into the homeless life," the Buddha voluntarily abandoned his wife and infant son, while Patacara exerted all her power to protect and keep her two babies, her husband, parents, and her brothers and sisters who, despite all her efforts, were torn from her. So I mulled over these differences, and also the deep similarity that guided these two in their paths.

Suddenly I felt the heat of sunlight on my chest, and noted that an hour had passed while I sat on my meditation cushion before the altar, with the book in my hands. Shaking my head, I closed the book, realizing that I had not meditated but had been sunk in contemplation the whole time. I had come close to my forebears in that India of thousands of years ago. Closing my eyes, I chanted in Pali, the sacred, literary language in which the original Buddhist canon, preserved for hundreds of years in an oral tradition, had been written down in the first century B.C.E. *"Namo tassa bhagavato, arahato, samma sambuddhasa."* Homage to the Buddha, the awakened one, the one perfectly enlightened by himself.

One night I went to sleep early and peacefully, and slept until 6 A.M. Lying in bed, rested, I felt in my body the desire to move, and I harked back to my regime for years when I had lived at Crystal's house: get up early, go out and ride my bicycle to Mountain View Cemetery, the same graveyard in which I had talked to Kwan Yin before my surgery. My bicycle stood in Jeannie's garage downstairs. My body wanted to try this again today. I dressed and went down the steps out into the fresh morning air to get my red bike. Squeezing the tires, I found them a bit mushy, but rideable. I got on the bike and started out, pedaling slowly, getting used to the motion. Few cars passed me on the side streets as I rode up toward the cemetery. The air felt cool against my skin. Ahead of me, where the hills of Oakland began to ascend, I saw the pale pinks and yellows of the rising sun.

Entering the big gates of the cemetery, I coasted past the pond where I had seen baby ducklings swimming in a line behind their mother two springs ago, and pedaled up the long central avenue under the huge old oaks and magnolia trees. All was still, cool, and clear, touched with pale radiance, this contained world seemingly trembling in anticipation of the light that would soon burst upon it. I rode steadily, looking around me, seeing a stray cat seated near a bush where kind people often left food, seeing the graves like mushrooms poking up from the grass, the land rising hill upon grave-studded hill to the rounded summit.

I had begun to sweat, and did not attempt the steeper inclines; instead I coasted down a long curving drive and came to the green slope where I had walked before my surgery. That had been less than a year ago. Surely Kwan Yin had been present. Now as I rode downhill I imagined glimpsing her, a woman in a flowing robe with an ornate headdress; I envisioned her simply there, standing humbly at the end of the blacktop drive, holding the vial of the liquid of compassion before her. She would not greet me, perhaps not even look at me, but simply show herself to me: yes, here I am, I exist. I smiled, seeing the empty drive. It curved down past the children's section, where grieving parents had left balloons and teddy bears and pinwheels on the little graves. And silently I chanted to Kwan Yin, *"Namo Guan-Shih-Yin pusa."* Homage to you, Kwan Yin bodhisattva who hears the cries of the world.

I circled the pond in the cool morning air as the sun rose higher, showering golden light on the trees, and I felt my aliveness with piercing happiness. Then as I headed back toward the entrance, I saw something move up ahead. This was not a stray cat but a larger animal, its coat deep red, with a great fluffy flag of a tail waving behind it. The fox crossed the blacktop, turning its pointed snout to glance in my direction, and trotted uphill among the graves. I took a deep, delighted breath, feeling blessed.

At home, upstairs in my bedroom, I found space between my bed and the door to do some yoga stretches, feeling my body relax, and remembered, yes, this is what I had done every morning, before cancer.

Then I sat down at my altar. After lighting candles and incense and ringing the bell to begin, I "took refuge" in the enlightened mind, in the way leading to it, and in all those who walked this path with me: I chanted, *"Buddham saranam gacchami* (I take refuge in the Buddha). *Dhammam saranam gacchami* (I take refuge in the Dharma). *Sangham saranam gacchami* (I take refuge in the Sangha)." I repeated the chant three times.

This morning I left the thick volume of the *Majjima Nikaya* unopened. Easily I slipped into attending to the breath, observing the slow inhalation and exhalation, feeling the vigor awakened in my body by the earlier exercise.

When half an hour had passed, I rang the bell, snuffed the candles, put away the book, and looked up at the bright-patterned curtains, which were suffused with sunlight. The day had begun.

17

Look Straight Ahead

Green leaves or fallen leaves
become one—
in the flowering snow.
Chiyo-ni

IN JUST A MONTH I would arrive at the anniversary of my surgery, and somewhere around that time I would have to undergo a colonoscopy, the test to determine whether the cancer had returned to my intestines. That future event began to exert its influence. The anxiety built, as powerful and capricious as if it had a life of its own, independent of me. I did everything not to fuel it, and yet it was there, like a ring in an animal's nose jerking it forward to a dreaded destination.

I began to awaken at four each morning and lie in bed unable to fall asleep again, my body tense. I had been calling Highland Hospital for days, trying to set up the appointment for the colonoscopy without success, and each day of missed communications increased my anxiety. If the test showed my intestine to be free of cancer, I could begin my life again. But there was a chance that a new growth would be found. Would it be small and easily removed? And if not, then what? More chemo? More surgery?

The apartment lay in stillness now in this middle of the night. Streetlight glow spilled filmy radiance through the window curtains. In the kitchen the refrigerator motor began to hum. How would I manage having cancer in these two small rooms, where I had not yet found a way to be comfortable? How could I tell my absent roommate Jeannie that she would be living with someone who might be very ill?

During the day, my concentration began to be affected by my dread.

I sat in my little study looking at the suggestions from writers and spiritual-teacher friends on my book, confused about how to benefit from their insights.

At the cancer support group, Rick Fields told us he was feeling overwhelmed. Wearing his usual rumpled jeans and casual jacket, he sat talking earnestly, looking around at each of our faces. At the *Yoga Journal*, where he was the editor, his colleagues were pressuring him to identify himself as a cancer patient in his next editorial, but Rick was not at all sure he wanted to come out publicly in that way. He spoke of stresses in his love relationship, and the physical difficulties attendant on the chemotherapy he was taking. And in the midst of all this he was trying to write a novel. "I don't want to give up anything!" he announced, sitting up straight with the warrior's determination that had kept him so passionately in life until now. Then he looked across the room at Rick Kohn, his friend and fellow Buddhist scholar, who had just told us that his own cancer had returned. "I'm so worried about him," Rick Fields confessed, and suddenly he was crying. "I want to fix it!" Along with most others in the room, I was crying too.

To end our session we rang the bell and sat in silence. On this day we pulled our chairs closer to clasp hands. I closed my eyes and let the bell's pure voice vibrate in my chest, and all that had been expressed settled in that sound. Yes, this is what is. I could feel that each of us, at least for this moment, accepted the reality of our compromised, perhaps dying, bodies; that we were willing to be with each other and ourselves in a kindly way, and to find peace in that.

Coming home, I saw Jeannie's truck parked in the garage, and as I climbed the stairs I heard her playing the upright piano in her room. In the kitchen I stood looking at the windowsill over the sink, where several of her small sculptures rested—male and female torsos molded in clay, sensitive and erotic. I liked living among Jeannie's sculptures, which reminded me of touch, of tenderness. At the center of the windowsill stood the little brown statue of Kwan Yin that I had placed there. Her robe swayed to the side as if blown by the sea wind, and I had curled seaweed and shells around her.

Jeannie rarely played her piano; I was sure she did not know that I had arrived home and could hear her. I sat down in a chair at the kitchen table, closed my eyes, and listened. The notes rose and cascaded in no predictable order. A theme emerged, and she followed it for a time, thoughtfully, then went in another direction, building a counter voice. It was as if she were talking to herself, mulling over a thought, exploring a feeling. Listening, I began to share her happiness in the playing, and I gave myself more fully to the sound.

When she stopped, the silence in the apartment was alive with the vibrance of her music. Opening my eyes I saw the little brown Kwan Yin limned with afternoon light. And I felt a joyful surrender in myself.

I was still weak, still recovering from the chemo. Each week I went to get acupuncture treatments, the chiropractor worked to release my whiplashed neck, and I walked carefully on my swollen ankle. Each morning I sat at my altar and, after reading a *sutta* in the *Majjima Nikaya,* I meditated, sometimes peacefully, more often now finding anxiety in myself. When that happened, I meditated by observing the anxiety. October progressed day by day toward the colonoscopy, which had finally been scheduled. I decided that on the night of the test I would have a dancing party, to which I would invite the people who had been most supportive of me over the preceding year. Jane, one of the Wandering Menstruals, who had a large comfortable home, offered her living room for the party. I love to dance, and even when I had been most depleted, if I found myself at an event where people were dancing, I always went past my lethargy and was able to dance with great pleasure. So it made sense to celebrate my freedom from cancer that way. But what if the news was bad? Well, then it would be a different kind of party, where I would ask my friends to sit down with me and ponder the challenge ahead. And *then* perhaps we might still get up and dance! It might be even more important to dance if the news were bad.

A further challenge leaped up at me. Crystal had found a tenant to live in the two rooms that had been my study and the living room. The woman renting the rooms was new to the community, and on the Saturday before my colonoscopy, Crystal had planned a potluck to welcome her and introduce her to friends. Now Crystal invited me to come to this party. My heart sank.

The weekend before the party, Crystal and I decided to spend some time together, and drove up to Jenner, on the Northern California coast, where a friend owned land and a trailer in which we could stay overnight. We spent Saturday at the cold, foggy beach, where a flock of pelicans careened through the air and then plunged one by one down into the surf to fish. We walked farther down the sand to watch the seals playing at the water's edge, lifting glistening dark heads to look around, and then disappearing under the foamy waves. After cooking dinner at the trailer, we sat outside looking up at a huge black sky full of stars. When we came inside, I lit the kerosene lamp and Crystal put a tape in the small tape player. From it issued the voice of Pema Chodron and we sat down on opposite sides of the dining table to listen.

During our years together, Crystal had attended retreats with me several times at Dhamma Dena, and at home she went periodically to a Zen priest for counseling, but her major discipline had been yoga and exercise. Now since my moving out, she told me, she had begun listening to tapes by Pema, becoming more interested in Buddhist perspectives. Both of us hoped that Pema's thoughts on how to meet hostility and suffering could help us in our efforts to salvage a friendship from the ruins of our love relationship.

The next morning, amazingly, perhaps because we were in this little trailer on the hillside above the ocean, far from the city and our former life together, we began to talk about the cancer time, each of us telling what it had been like for her at its worst. Perhaps I had left my anger and sorrow temporarily on the misty beach, for I was able to hear how very confused and overburdened Crystal had felt, how she could not control her reactions to me, and how sometimes she had not known how to ask for help. Then she felt that my friends had overlooked all the actual labor she was performing and simply blamed her for what she had not been able to do. She felt I had blamed her also. In return, I told her how I had felt after each painful encounter with her, and how my distrust of her had grown until one afternoon when I had been sleeping on the couch, and she came in from the kitchen carrying a knife, I had actually imagined that she would stab me to death. I had known that in my weakness I would not be able to defend myself. Crystal was horrified, hearing this, but I told her I had become convinced that, whether she was conscious of it or not, she had wanted to get rid of me. We talked about the awful distortion in both of our perspectives, mine from illness and the drugs, hers from panic and the pressure of trying to keep up with my care while living her own life.

Both of us cried, holding hands across the little table in the trailer.

Softened by this opening, during our drive back to Oakland I let her persuade me to come to the housewarming party; I agreed to put in an appearance for Crystal's sake, to show her friends that we were not enemies now. And privately, I vowed to simply let my feelings on that day be what they were.

Two days later, back in my rooms at Jeannie's house, while I was struggling with a jammed computer, I began to cry heartbrokenly. I went in the bedroom and lay on the bed and gave up to this grieving, sobbing without thoughts. Later, I felt so raw that I did not want to go out on the street. I knew that a traumatic event gets encoded in the body and has to work its way out, in its own time. The anniversary of my surgery would arrive in a few days. I woke often at night; during the day I felt vulnerable and shaky.

With weird irony, Crystal's party for her new roommate had been scheduled for the actual date the year before when I had been operated on. I determined not to go alone, and asked my good friend Annie if she would accompany me. Annie concocted a plan: we would meet earlier at my house to do some sort of ceremony to commemorate the day. We'd go to Crystal's party just long enough to meet the new roommate and be reasonably gracious, then we would escape to a movie. (Annie, a filmmaker, never lost an opportunity to see a film.)

The Saturday came, and I sat at my little altar alone. Annie lay in the bed behind me, felled by a bad cold, napping in order to be able to go on with our plan. The street outside my windows was fairly quiet; the twin toddlers were playing peacefully on their porch.

I rang the bell and took refuge, and then I began to do the *metta*, or loving-kindness, practice. The goal of the loving-kindness practice is to promote a vital, outflowing current from the meditator to all life, to teach us not to separate ourselves from the rest of humanity. The attitude to be cultivated was expressed by the Buddha: "As a mother, even at the risk of her own life, protects and loves her child, her only child, so let [us] cultivate love without measure toward the whole world, above, below and around, unstinted, unmixed with any feeling of differing or opposing interests." We are asked to honor our strong connection with the beings around us and our responsibility to meet each of them with an open heart.

To begin, I visualized myself as if I were seated before me, and I sent loving-kindness to myself. I imagined the people closest to me, opened my heart, and sent love to them. Then I saw Crystal there before me: I acknowledged my complicated, unresolved feelings for her, and remembered our recent candor in the trailer. Could I open my heart to her? Could I send positive loving thoughts to her? I imagined Crystal at her most fragile, realizing once again how terrifying my illness had been for her, and my heart filled with love. "May you be free from enmity," I wished her. "May you be free from grief and disease. May you be happy." Then I imagined her new roommate, whom I had not yet met—a faceless woman, to whom I sent loving-kindness. Widening my scope, I sent warm feelings to every being in my neighborhood, in the city of Oakland, and then in the United States, the world, and the universe. I ended by once again focusing loving energy on myself, feeling strongly centered now.

Annie snored softly in the bed behind me. I looked at the card she had brought me, a card from the Tarot deck that she had pulled for me that morning: the four of disks. The description spoke of making a sanctuary, a place of safety to retreat to in order to do inner work. I was grateful for Annie's caring, her concern that I hold steady and protect myself.

Then I found myself thinking about that coming Tuesday when I would go to Highland for the colonoscopy. Sitting at my altar watching the candle flames flicker, the incense send up a lazy curl of fragrant smoke, I felt strongly in myself that whatever would happen on Tuesday, I would still be the same person afterwards—that in a sense, the outcome did not matter, since I would just continue to live each moment of my life anyway, whether I were living it as a cancer patient or a healthy person.

I had been reading some Japanese poems on death. One of them I had copied and put on my altar. Now I picked up the little sheet of paper and read:

> Look straight ahead. What's there?
> If you see it as it is
> You will never err.

A Zen monk named Bassui Tokusho had composed that. Always the same message: be awake for what is happening right now. Look straight ahead, even at the moment of death.

I took a deep breath, hearing the squeal of a car peeling rubber at the corner, seeing the bright curtains tremble in a faint breeze, feeling the weight of my body on my cushion, I closed my eyes and turned my attention to the sensations of my sitting body.

Later Annie parked her car on the street, and we got out. I looked up at the yellow frame house. Crystal and I had always driven into the driveway and entered through the back door. Only strangers, students, visitors, came to the front. I stood on the sidewalk looking up the brick steps to the porch, realizing I was a visitor now, just another guest invited to this party. I wanted to turn and run.

But I followed Annie up the steps. Our ring was answered by a short woman with a sweet round face. "I'm Vivian," she said, and shook our hands. I realized she was the new roommate. When I told her my name, her eyes widened a bit and she nodded. She laughed uncomfortably. "Welcome to your former space." I found myself smiling, wanting to put her at ease.

Then I stepped inside and looked around, seeing a bed where my desk had been, a rack of shelves where our couch had sat. The furniture and objects hovered before me, as if superimposed on those other two rooms that remained just as they had been when I had worked there each day and taught my classes. I suffered an awful inner slippage, seeing both pictures vividly and then knowing that the actual physical reality was this visible one, of Vivian's counter and computer in the living room, her bed and chairs and bureau, and her pictures newly hung on the wall. *My* rooms hovered ghostlike behind this scene, pulling at my heart.

Annie led me into the kitchen, where we could hear the chatter of women's voices. We set down food we had brought, and began to talk with the other guests. Crystal, busy being hostess, greeted us briefly. I listened to the conversation, putting in a word now and then, enjoying the people and interested in their opinions. But another parallel consciousness existed simultaneously in me. I was feeling the familiar space of these rooms, recognizing it: this was my house, my rooms—to be quiet and comfortable in, to work in. Silently I raged: *I should be here.* Why did I have to move out?!

Half an hour later, we managed to leave. As we drove away I sat in locked silence. "Do you want to scream?" Annie asked. I would not have thought of that. I decided to try it, letting out a howl that left me shaking.

Abruptly I realized how far I had been pulled away from the loving-kindness I had experienced earlier. I saw how my feelings for Crystal gyrated wildly, spinning me away from my center. As we drove through the crowded streets to the movie, I felt my anger like fire in my veins, shielding me from sadness.

In the trinity of greed, hatred, and delusion—those human tendencies that in Buddhism drive the great wheel of becoming—my most conscious challenge is hatred or ill will. When I am hurt, anger rises in me. Typically I have acted on that anger by withdrawing my energy and hardening my heart, but sometimes by striking out with impatience or sarcasm at the one who frightened or criticized me. Only recently have I begun to learn to hold still: not to act but simply to be with my anger, and always that brings me to the hurt feelings that occasioned it. Sometimes now I am able to let the anger go and stay with the original response, admitting my vulnerability.

Of course I know the childhood antecedents of this in myself, how the angry withdrawal helped me survive in dangerous family situations. But I wonder how much of our behavior can be attributed to our experiences, and how big a part temperament or some kind of original nature plays in us. If we believe that something of us returns, life after life, then we may bring tendencies with us that triumph over our conditioning. I think of Ruth Denison, her childhood in a little Prussian village, where her teachers referred to her as the "golden *mitte*," the golden center, for her capacity to bring balance to any situation. "I had no trouble with anger," Ruth told me.

In her twenties, having survived her war experience, Ruth was not broken or embittered. She was able to return to normal life, become a teacher again, come to this country, marry. And when her husband took her to Burma to study with the great Burmese meditation master U Ba Khin, she was ready. "I had no anger, no need for revenge. These are good karmic forces for the spiritual path."

Another Buddhist teacher, the Venerable Ayya Khema, a German Jew, had been put in a concentration camp with her family as a child and had seen her father die there, yet she too bore no rancor. She went regularly to Germany to teach, and even established a meditation center there.

As I pondered my anger at Crystal, I saw that anger was a way to avoid the real import of Vivian's party. Standing in that living room, I had been presented with the truth: that my shared life with Crystal was over. The pain of that realization came strongly to me in the days that followed.

But it was soon eclipsed by the enormous surge of anxiety running like an electric current through me as the day of the colonoscopy approached. Just under the surface of my mind lay the awareness that in a few days' time, my fate would be decided.

Even in the midst of this grim anticipation there came moments of huge relief. The day after Crystal's party brought another anniversary. I awoke to a quiet apartment, got up to make tea, and came back to sit in bed, watching the light begin to illuminate the rainbow curtains. My cat, who had come to join me a month ago, curled up on my legs and went to sleep.

Sipping my tea, I remembered where I had been last year on this day: Highland Hospital, seventh floor, in that noisy room, the tube down my nose and throat, IV needle in my hand, and an eight-inch gash in my stomach. I remembered sliding in and out of consciousness, struggling to *be there* through the morphine haze. My friends. And the deep rich voices of the Webb Sisters singing...*I once was lost, but now I'm found; was blind but now I see....*

I took a deep breath, looking around my little room with its books, green plants, and altar. The sun brightened the curtains now, and outside in the street some bicyclists shifted gears and talked with each other, their voices growing louder and then drifting away. I filled my lungs with cool morning air. And with sudden delight I thought, *I'm alive!*

Later that day, Crystal called to say she wanted to take me to the hospital on Tuesday. I told her my reaction to her party, and we talked briefly about the circumstances of my moving out. Crystal maintained that there had been other options, that I had acted hastily. We argued a bit, and when I put down the phone I stood thinking. It seemed as if during that hard time, each of us had been swept up into doing things she didn't want to do and resenting that. Unhappily, I wondered how I could take full responsibility for my part. Would we ever be able to clarify what had happened between us?

On Monday evening, as directed, I began to drink the gallon of "Golightly" that would clean out my intestines for the coming test, and prepared for a night of frequent visits to the bathroom. Each time, awakened by my grumbling gut, I crawled out of bed, trying not to disturb the

cat, who slept peacefully on Sandy's outspread down-filled coat. Returning, I crawled wearily under the covers, feeling a headache coming on.

In the pale morning light I stood in the kitchen and looked at the little brown statue poised on the windowsill. "Do me a favor, Kwan Yin,"
I said. "Make it turn out okay." No response. I went back to my room to
dress, remembering my petition to Kwan Yin last year in the graveyard
and how the answer had finally come from myself. This morning my
head ached and I felt weak, dreading the coming ordeal. I would have to
do without the equanimity; just being miserable would have to suffice.

Crystal was waiting for me at the curb in front of the apartment house,
in the little gray Toyota we had owned together. "How're you holding
up?" she asked as I fastened my seat belt. "Groan," I answered. "I'll stay
with you in the waiting room," Crystal reassured me. As we could not
know when the test would be over, I had made arrangements for Sandy
Butler to pick me up afterwards.

As we drove out the highway I could see the great gray wedge of the
hospital looming above the neighborhood. How I wished I were on my
way anywhere but there. I checked myself: Sandy, stay present.

On the third floor, we headed for the Gastro-Intestinal Lab. I could see
Bill Shanks at the other end of the corridor, clipboard in hand, leaning
over a seated oncology patient. I wanted to shout at him, to receive some
of his constant warmth. Save me, Bill!

But we entered the G.I. lab, where the nurse took my blood pressure
and temperature, and then sent us back to the waiting room. Crystal and
I sat next to each other, trying to ignore the abrasive talk show on the television. A family of four sat with us, their eyes on the set. Crystal looked
tired; she found it hard to get up so early in the morning, I knew, and I
realized what an effort it must have been for her to make this gesture.

"I appreciate your bringing me," I told her. "I hope it won't be too
many hours till they take me in."

Crystal squeezed my arm. "It's okay. I'm here for as long as it takes."

Surprisingly soon the nurse came to get me. "Your friend can't come
with you," she said. "Sorry." I turned back to Crystal. "Well…" She gave
me a hug. "Good luck. Will you call me as soon as you know?" And I
watched her walk toward the elevator.

I'm beset by the urge to fictionalize, to invent *Saturday-Evening-Post*
moments. Like this: As I follow the nurse toward the G.I. entrance,

Crystal comes back. She grabs my hand, and I see her blue eyes frightened for me, and caring. "I'm praying that it'll be okay," she says urgently. No, there was no second thought, no rush of emotion. The elevator door closed behind Crystal's erect back, her wavy gray hair.

What is this impulse to lie? I'm still wanting, I guess, to avoid the way it really was. Crystal left. The nurse took me into a room filled with shiny chrome equipment and three gurneys, two of which were occupied. She told me to take off my clothes, put on the hospital gown and lie down on the gurney to wait until the doctors were ready for me. I obeyed.

For three hours I lay on the gurney, woozy from not eating and shitting all night, dozing when I could. The only diversion—mildly interesting and also annoying—was the doctor's conversation with one of the nurses. In a loud voice he chronicled his recent trip to Rome, concentrating especially on the meals he had eaten. As he described these dinners from pasta to fruit and cheese, I lay listening, thinking on the one hand that this recital was rather insensitive in the setting of a county hospital in which most of those within earshot might never get farther from home than Sacramento, and on the other hand trying to visualize each dish as he described it. My mind ran on as I wondered if he had stopped work to give his travelogue, and thus slowed down the process for all concerned, especially me.

Three hours is a long time to lie on a gurney in a cold room. I resorted to concentrating on my breath, following it in and out, in and out, connecting as best as I could to my body.

Finally the nurse came to wheel me inside, into a darkened room with a TV monitor hung above the spot where she parked my gurney. The doctor came in, reading my chart, and asked me a few questions while the nurse gave me two shots. "One's to deal with pain," the doctor explained, "the other for anxiety." We waited again, this time for the drugs to take hold.

Of the doctor I remember an earnest face and thinning hair, and an impatient, authoritative voice. When I was sufficiently woozy and lying on my back, the doctor carefully inserted the tube in my anus, talking all the while about what he was doing at each moment. The TV monitor began to blink and everyone turned to it. Then there appeared, in lurid color, my intestine, seen from the inside, a shiny pink tube with twists and folds. The doctor jiggled the mini camera up through every inch of this tube, doing a running commentary as he went. I was mesmerized by the vision of my innards, and all my energy in my exceedingly groggy state went into staring at the screen. Somewhere outside my dim tent of attention I could hear the doctor's voice describing what he saw.

"No polyps. No suspicious growths." Did that mean…?

And then he was removing the tube. I realized he was looking me in the face, and I tried to concentrate on what he was saying to me. "You're clear. You're all clear."

I hovered in a strange half-world, not really grasping his meaning.

Back in the lighted room, in a curtained cubicle, the nurse stayed with me, asking me how I felt. I saw the numbers on the blood pressure machine. Fifty-five over twenty-two. Thinking this must be an error, I joked to the nurse, "I'm dead." But it wasn't a joke. "The drugs cause your blood pressure to drop severely," she explained. "You'll be okay in a little while."

An hour later Sandy Butler took me out into the sunshine of a clear autumn day. When I had told her the news, we shrieked and hugged, but there was an unreality to it. More real were the neat houses sparkling in the sun, Sandy's warm excited voice repeating, "Mazel tov!" and the springy, light feel of my body as we walked up the hill to her car.

In the car on our way to eat at a favorite Chinese restaurant I sat tensely, uncertain what exactly had transpired. Then, at the Little Shin Shin, I applied myself to the spinach-tofu soup, so soothing to my empty stomach. I could feel my body settle a little, coming back into itself. As we ate the main dishes laced with garlic, Sandy and I chattered. At times I would stop talking and eating and feel a wave of tension leave my body, as I breathed out—a loosening—and would look up to see Sandy smiling encouragingly at me, as if to say, "Yes, it *is* real."

At a nearby coffeehouse, we bought drinks and a slice of cake to share, and drove the few blocks to the Mountain View cemetery. Sitting on a hillside among the graves, I looked at the sunlight gilding the leaves of the great spreading trees and the grass so intensely, moistly green under the shade. We ate and drank, and talked of many things—about the book party I would give next year to celebrate the publication of *Opening the Lotus*, about a possible trip to Ireland, and about a dream I had had for years of going to the Okefenokee Swamp in Florida to work with the manatees, large aquatic mammals sometimes referred to as sea cows because of their lumbering, gentle demeanor; they are now endangered by the housing developments and boats on the waterways they inhabit. I was telling Sandy about the project to map the location of individual manatees in the shallow coastal waters so that their habitat can be protected, when I felt another level of tension leave me, as if a tight garment had loosened and fallen away.

Sandy grinned at me. "I promise you, when you settle down, I'll help you plan the rest of your life!" We laughed again about how much pleasure Sandy took in planning.

That evening the dancing party seemed lifted up on a wave of elation. I taped a sign to the door announcing that this was "Liberation Tuesday," so that each guest would know the result before she entered. Then I let myself move fully into the happiness and relief that all of us felt. My friends arrived bearing champagne, a chocolate mousse pie, and bouquets of flowers. Everyone wanted to hug me and tell me how glad she was about the news. Then we sat in a circle, and I told the story of my day, introduced each of the women, and described how she had participated in my healing. When it came time to tell about Crystal, I hesitated, impaled on the sword of my ambivalence. I had invited her to the party because she had been centrally present in the experience of this year, but my feelings for her shifted so dramatically—from love to resentment and back again—that it was hard to think of how to thank her. From a Buddhist perspective I might simply have honored her for the myriad ways in which she had helped me when I was most ill, and let go of our conflicts, the awful disagreements that had wracked us during those months. But I could not shake free of the residue of that struggle to wholeheartedly express my gratitude. Crystal sat on the floor among the other women, waiting, watching me with uncertain eyes. I floundered, gave in to defeat, and finally found something mild and neutral to say.

But that night nothing could dampen my happiness. Soon we got up to boogie. Gyrating to the music, I felt my body release yet another cape of tension. We shared our joy, all of us dancing together, at one point forming two lines down which each individual moved, even my friend in a wheelchair managing to dance with great abandon.

Later, back at Jeannie's place, I sat on my bed in the darkened room, hearing a car pass on the street below. I looked at the squares of windows, brighter than the surrounding darkness, the patterns of the curtains blurred. Below the windows my altar was lost in shadow. I imagined the faces of my treasured dead—my brother George, Maurine Stuart, Lex Hixon, my mother and father. George's presence felt strong in the room, as if he rejoiced with me, and I saw his gentle, sensitive face. It resembled the face of Lex Hixon, and as I visualized them, the two men merged into one being: a man who smiled at me, the luminous flower of his heart radiating light.

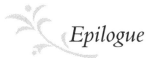

Epilogue

*The heart is always the place to go. Go home into your
heart, where there is warmth, appreciation, gratitude
and contentment.*

Ayya Khema

IT IS NOW ALMOST FIVE YEARS since the events in this book occurred.
Each year I have had a colonoscopy that showed no tumor or other
growth in my intestines. If there are cancer cells lurking in my body they
have not shown themselves yet, for which I am grateful. I find myself
grateful for many things just now, particularly the writing of this book,
which required me to return to and relive the most painful year of my
life, a process that was sometimes excruciating.

Why did I choose to do it? There was a moment, during one of my
hospitalizations, that persuaded me to write this book. That day the head
surgeon visited me. His name was Dr. Organ (no kidding) and he was a
large, brown-skinned, handsome man who radiated the kind of
confidence that comes from substantial accomplishment and recognition.
Dr. Organ was interested in my being a writer, and we discussed the books
on the table next to my bed. As I explained to him what each was about,
I felt a little embarrassed: would he think I was morbid in my literary
tastes, given my condition? Yet Dr. Organ listened with great interest.

When he had left the room and I was alone again, I looked at the
books I had brought with me to the hospital. Author Nan Shin explored,
among other things, her experience of ovarian cancer in her luminous-
ly written *Diary of a Zen Nun;* Isabel Allende chronicled the slow dying
of her daughter in *Paula;* Audre Lorde, African-American lesbian poet-
warrior, wrote of her struggle with liver cancer in *A Burst of Light.* A visiting friend, seeing this small angst-ridden library, had asked me, "Why
would you want to read this stuff?!"

The answer was that I could stomach nothing but this vision that looked straight at death. I wanted to hear from those who had gone where I now found myself, and farther. I wanted to hear what thoughts they had, what they felt, whether they could meet their suffering bravely or if they crumpled before it, and if there was meaning in it for them. After my conversation with Dr. Organ, lifting these books and holding them, I thought, if I have this need, others must feel it too. And I realized that I would write about my encounter with cancer, drawing another tiny map of the territory to help the next woman or man who had to make this journey. As if to say, this is just how it is; someone else has walked this way.

During the writing of this book, besides the necessary revisiting of pain and loss, I began to view my spiritual practice in a way that I never had before. In the months of producing the book I have observed myself, sometimes with surprise, actually living my awareness with greater understanding than before.

The capacity to tolerate grief, loneliness, frustration, and anger—to see those conditions as mind-states that will pass—is developing in me. Returning into the cancer time, I saw myself experiencing the truth that even in the midst of intense suffering, life bubbles up, offering joy. I saw how quickly our feelings and ideas about things pass: for this hour I was despairing, then suddenly delight came, now I was anxious, now confident.... These mental states follow one upon the other endlessly. I saw that I watched them, participated in them, now and then wallowed in them, and finally let them go. Life continues to create itself and fall away: suffering returns, and then delight arrives; successive moments bring agony, peace, rapture. I learned not to imagine that any of these states would endure for very long. I did my best to tune in to the flow of phenomena, in which we are always in transit, our bodies changing, our emotions passing through a rainbow of feelings and thoughts; in which we are always inhabiting concepts and letting them go. I saw myself in the cancer months staying present to that flux.

Pema Chodron, in an early conversation about monasticism, said something that struck me. Monasticism removes so many of the props to our ego. Hair shorn, individuality hidden under the brown robe, and focus sharpened by the schedule of meditation, study, and work, a truly practicing nun or monk gets herself or himself out of the way. And then what is experienced? Beaming at me, Pema described the immense creativity expressed in the arising and falling away of phenomena in every moment. I got the impression that her perception of this was like watching a brilliantly rich and entertaining performance.

While I am nowhere near that condition of clarity and detachment, I have come to more gratitude for the amount of reality of which I *am* aware.

I also find myself wanting to offer comfort and kindness where I can. A few years ago the Charlotte Maxwell Complementary Clinic, where I had received excellent care, asked me to teach a writing workshop at a retreat for cancer patients. I readily accepted. The clinic had received a grant to pay all expenses for the participants in this retreat. Fifty cancer patients were bussed or drove to the hills of northern California for this three-day gathering. Among them were a large proportion of women of color—African American, Hispanic, Asian. Many of these women and the low-income white women would never have been able, on their own, to get out of the city to the relative luxury of gracious old residences and a large dining hall that served excellent food. It was a treat for them to be there, away from family responsibilities and jobs.

Many of the women were gravely ill, bald from chemo, walking slowly supported by canes or walkers. As I talked with these women, I realized a major effect of my own cancer: now I knew what it felt like to move slowly and with great effort while others strode easily past; to look at a plate of food and have my stomach begin to rise up into my throat; to exist in a vague, energyless state, feeling vulnerable to the physical world, weighed down and inadequate. Because of this knowledge I was comfortable with the women's illness and debility, able to see through the symptoms into the person who was always there, intact, as *I* had been at the worst moments. Before cancer, I had been frightened by illness, and had often pulled away to protect myself; now I understood that there was nothing to protect, and I found myself capable of being attentively present with each woman there.

The women who had chosen to attend my workshop joined me in a small lounge, where we settled on couches and comfortable chairs. I asked them to write a letter to their bodies, expressing what they thought and felt.

As the women wrote, I looked around the room. Here was an Indian woman with the short crewcut of someone coming back from chemo baldness, a young white woman who looked energetic and healthy, a snowy-haired old woman reclining on a couch, an African-American woman who I knew was an organizer as well as recipient of services, and others. Everyone bent to her task.

When I asked them to read their letters aloud, I could feel them pull back. Their faces told me that the words they had put on paper would be difficult to reveal to others. Finally one woman read her short letter, with her head down. "The loving, touching men are gone." She struggled to maintain composure as she went on, "the women and children are still here. They love us for who we are and just the way we are." Tears coursed down her face as she looked up at us in astonishment. "I didn't think I would *cry!*" she exclaimed.

For an instant I faltered. Had I made a mistake? Had I plunged these women into gratuitous suffering, for the sake of an exercise? It was a heart-stopping moment.

Then the African-American woman spoke from across the room. "It's good to let it out. Go ahead and cry." And she added, "I keep a journal. Every day I do this, and it helps me go on."

Heads nodded.

Every woman in the room read, then, some expressing grief at their losses, some detailing their determined coping with the effects of disease and treatment. Each letter began *"Dear Body,"*

—I see that your salivary glands are not moistening the right side of your mouth since the radiation. Here, keep this water with you always…

—Yes, you're seventy years old now. It's not just the numbers but what happened four-and-a-half years ago when your cells kept dividing and you had surgery for breast and ovarian cancer. You recovered very well and didn't even cry until your hair fell out! Oh how vain we are!

—I do not like this body anymore…I used to feel sexy, attractive…. Now I feel no one is looking at me…. My body image, well what can I say? You have been chopped up so.

More tears were shed as the women read their letters. I realized that this expression, heavy as it felt in its rawness and honesty, came as a relief to everyone there, that it cleansed and lightened.

When I asked if the women's writings could appear in the clinic newsletter, they thought about the prospect, and then almost everyone in the room agreed to let her words be published. They understood how useful these expressions might be to other people enduring the trauma of serious illness. Just as I had sought out the words of Audre Lorde, Isabel Allende, and Nan Shin, these women knew the importance of communicating the truth of our experience.

This last year Kwan Yin lifted me up and sent me out into the world, as if to say, "Now make yourself useful." At the end of the writing of *Discovering Kwan Yin* when it was time to publicize that book, She Who Hears the Cries of the World instructed me, "Say yes to everything anyone asks you to do." I did so, and found myself leading meditation retreats introducing Kwan Yin's being and practices to people who sought them out, and drawing upon my years of training with Ruth Denison.

Many of the people who come to these retreats are caregivers, people who work as nurses, therapists, social workers, mothers, and teachers; people who give a great deal on a daily basis and receive very little in return. Kwan Yin offers them the opportunity to relax into compassionate energy, to engage in self-nurturing, and to renew their strength.

My cancer support group no longer meets. Speaking at the memorial service for Rick Fields, Rick Kohn articulated a truth about such groups. "On the one hand, it's great support, and you come to love the people," he said. "On the other, it's very sad, because they die." Many of the group members have passed on. Rick Kohn himself is now gravely ill. And there are other members whom I run into from time to time, who are in remission from their cancer, or cured. One particular woman, who was undergoing devastating radiation for throat cancer while in the group, I met one day at an event. She was vibrant and energetic, wholly returned to life. We reminisced about the meetings, about the two Ricks and our wonderful nurse-leader Jan, whom both of us saw as a bodhisattva. I knew the group had been a special conjunction of personalities coming together for a time and then disintegrating, and felt privileged to have participated in it.

After I quit the chemo, four years ago, gradually over the ensuing weeks and months my body recovered from the assault of the poisons. I worked at getting well, building strength, hoping my damaged tissues would repair themselves. But I have found that some of the effects of the chemotherapy still remain with me. I have almost no sense of smell, and my ability to taste has been diminished. I assume these changes are permanent, and I miss my former keen capacity to enjoy odors and tastes.

There is a deeper change. My identification with my body is seriously compromised. I have known its malfunction, its weakness; I have come close to losing this body to death. I had had experience in meditation of the impermanence of my physical self and its existence as flux, as a dance of energy. But now I sometimes perceive myself in quite ordinary social situations not as a solid entity but as a sheet of light passing through, or as an unfocused vibration hovering in the scene.

In my spiritual practice I plod slowly along on the road to bare attention, or "choiceless awareness." I like to listen to a song by Heng Yin, an American-born Buddhist nun. Called "Great Is the Joy," the song evokes her feelings about the practice. One line says, "The sea of suffering is deep and wide [but] a turn of the head is the other side." That always reminds me that liberation is with us, that with one sideways glance one may find oneself transported across the waters to the "other shore" of freedom from suffering.

Certainly, joy is available to me in many ways. For the turn of the millennium I journeyed south to Dhamma Dena, to come home into the Dharma-stream sustained by Ruth Denison. She was her usual indomitable self, even though her husband Henry was experiencing the last process of his dying in a house not far from the meditation hall. Henry was attended by Dharma students and by Ruth, whenever she could take time from the retreat to visit him. For forty years a strong bond had held them together: Henry was the person who had taken Ruth to Burma and introduced her to her teacher U Ba Khin, and she would always be loyal to him in gratitude for that priceless gift.

On December 31, 1999, the meditation hall was full of people who had come to escape the millennium "Y2K" hysteria, to experience a sane, peaceful transition into the new year. We had rested an hour or two after the evening meal, put on our most festive casual clothes, and arrived at the meditation hall to find our pillows arranged in a circle so that we could all face each other. To begin, Ruth led the *Namo tassa* chant to the Buddha, and then she asked me to introduce a prayer and meditation that we would share with people in every part of the globe. The notice

I had received about this global prayer and meditation had projected that for New Year's Eve 2000, over a billion people from all over the world would engage in a few moments of prayer or meditation for world peace. Once again we would acknowledge our interdependence with all life.

As our participation in this global effort, Ruth led a *metta* meditation, sending loving-kindness to all beings in the universe. Then she asked us to stand up and improvised a dance. The night before, in her Dharma talk, she had explained the Eightfold Noble Path to enlightenment, dividing it into the usual three parts—*sila* (ethical conduct), *samadhi* (concentration), and *panna* (wisdom). Tonight she began to chant the three words, leading us in a sideways circle dance. *"Sila, samadhi, panna,"* we chanted as we sidestepped and dipped, and for some reason everyone seemed delighted. I felt the joy in movement, and in the meaning of the words. I was so glad to be alive and to be here once again at Dhamma Dena. "Be mindful of your beautiful selves," Ruth told us. "Know what you are doing." She swung out in a slow pirouette, lifting her hands as if inviting the celestial beings to join us.

It reminded me of the many New Year's Eves I had spent here. Now Ruth, at age seventy-seven, seemed as agile and spontaneous as when I first knew her, animated by her passion to invite us to the Dharma.

After the dancing, Ruth sent us back to sit on our pillows and brought out a large bag of used ribbons and gift wrappings. Approaching a rather dour, baldheaded man, she draped curled ribbons across his pate and taped them on to create a wacky holiday hat. Others rose to help her, and soon everyone was being decorated in more or less whimsical fashion. I found myself among the milliners, extracting bright paper from the bag, leaning over a seated meditator to shape yet another outrageous creation. I realized that this willingness to participate so fully in an innocent, silly activity had developed in me after the cancer. Before, I might have sat locked in embarrassment or disapproval.

As midnight approached Ruth brought the big bell shaped like a stew pot to the center of the meditation hall. We would ring the bell 108 times, she announced. She would begin, and after ten strikes someone else would take his or her turn. At the end of each set of ten strikes, we were to call out some aspect of ourselves that we would like to get rid of.

This is a traditional practice followed in the Zen tradition, based on the thirty-six delusions as they are perceived in the past, present, and future;

the number can refer also to the 108 forms of enlightenment detailed in the Heart Sutra: one can imagine that as each negative quality is called out, a door to enlightenment is opened.

Everyone gathered around the bell, and the ringing began.

While we counted together, I thought of my failures in the preceding year, most particularly my inability to relate steadily and compassionately with Crystal. We had worked at repairing the relationship and had experienced much forgiveness, but finally I had come to understand that I could never return to the partnership in a way that would be wholesome for her and for me. I was not a bodhisattva, motivated by endless compassion: I was a flawed person who had been wounded in a relationship, and could not completely free myself from that legacy. With the ringing of the bell, I offered up my weakness, my selfishness, and anger, and as each stroke fell into silence I vowed to strive to be more aware of my own behavior in the coming year, to open into more spaciousness. After the hundredth ring, Ruth took the striker and tolled the final eight tones to bring in the year 2000.

I looked around at the radiant faces of my Dharma-mates and realized that we had entered the twenty-first century together, reinforcing the values of the Buddha, Dharma, and Sangha once again, committing ourselves to the path of liberation.

The evening ended with a meditation led by Ruth, to renew our dedication to mindfulness of the body and to officially welcome the New Year.

I came out into the night, walked halfway between the meditation hall and the eating hall and stood among the creosote and desert sage bushes looking upward. The sky wheeled like a carousel above me, spinning arrows and dippers and great bright globes—all unexpectedly big and seeming very close. The sky dominated with its limitless depth and fierce light, with very little competition from below; only a few porch lights and window squares were visible out across the flat black desert. Dhamma Dena's Christmas lights along the roof of the meditation hall gave off a feeble caterpillar glow. The stars seemed to strut and sail about, advertising their transcendence. It was no wonder that the ancients had made up stories about them: they clanged with authority above the dust-laden desert.

I gazed upward, neck craned back, feeling my mind and heart, loves and griefs sucked out into this circus of a sky. If I were not shivering already, I might have lain down on the sandy soil and surrendered to this wild, ancient dance.

Taking a deep breath of cold night air, I turned to walk back to Samadhi House, where I was ensconced in a tiny room like a nun's cell. I took stock of my life. I was learning to be alone in the world, to take full responsibility for myself. I had moved again, into a new place where I felt I had entered a new life. At age sixty-three, I had a heightened sense of the brevity of the time ahead of me, and that unburdened me of much baggage from the past. There were some books I wanted to write, some places on the globe I wanted to visit. I hoped to stay as healthy as I was for many years to come. My heart was filled with gratitude for Ruth Denison and her teachings, for this place called Dhamma Dena, for the cancer that had taught me so much, and for its absence now. I remembered a moment the day before: During the holiday retreats, at the end of each morning session, Ruth played a portion of a tape of Handel's Messiah sung in English. The day before, in this beautiful music that commemorated the coming of the light in the darkness of winter, the soloist sang, "I know that my redeemer liveth," and tears began to stream down my face, for I understood the message for me, the knowledge of that luminous ground that underlies our lives and resides deep in each of us. My redeemer is that consciousness, that great ground of being into which we continually disappear and are continually reborn.

Now in the black spangled desert night, at this place of effort and struggle, risk and safety I realized that my life was finite and precious, and that if the cancer returned I would try to meet it in the spirit of the Zen teacher Maurine Stuart—not make a move to avoid it. And perhaps come to the place in myself where I could wholeheartedly speak the words of Sono, ancient Shin Buddhist devotee, who said, "Thanks for everything. I have no complaints whatsoever."

I dedicate the merit of this book to all those suffering from disease and facing death, to Henry Denison in his passing, to my teacher Ruth Denison in her growing older, and to all creatures, human, animal, and in whatever other configurations they may exist. May we experience peace and well-being. May we be free from grief and fear. May we be happy.

Other Titles by Wisdom Publications

LESSONS FROM THE DYING
Rodney Smith

"[This is] a book that, page for page, word for word, is one of the best 'meaning of life' books around, rivaling Victor Frankl's classic *Man's Search for Meaning* in power and insight and surpassing it in depth. Complementing his many anecdotes of personal confrontations with death, Smith analyzes why and how we often short-change ourselves emotionally, and at the end of each chapter, he offers exercises for cultivating human wholeness. There are books about death and grieving. This is a book about transforming life."—Amazon.com

224 pages, ISBN 0-86171-140-8, $16.95

Books on Meditation

MINDFULNESS IN PLAIN ENGLISH
Henepola Gunaratana

"One of the best nuts-and-bolts meditation manuals.... If you'd like to learn the practice of meditation, you can't do better."
—Amazon.com

"A masterpiece. I cannot recommend it highly enough."
—Jon Kabat-Zinn, author of *Wherever You Go, There You Are*

208 pages, ISBN 0-86171-064-9, $14.95

JOURNEY TO THE CENTER
A MEDITATION WORKBOOK
Matthew Flickstein
Foreword by Bhante Gunaratana

"The workbook format makes the meditations easy to follow, simple to do, and very effective. Flickstein leads readers to uncover unconscious memories, discover new, positive ideas, and open the way to change.... *Journey to the Center* is a guide to successful living."—*New Age Retailer*

224 pages, ISBN 0-86171-141-6, $15.95

HOW TO MEDITATE
A PRACTICAL GUIDE
Kathleen McDonald

"An excellent introduction...refreshingly readable...clarity without over-simplification."—*Buddhist Studies Review*

224 pages, ISBN 0-86171-009-6, $14.95

WISDOM ENERGY
BASIC BUDDHIST TEACHINGS—TWENTY-FIFTH ANNIVERSARY EDITION
Lama Yeshe and Lama Zopa Rinpoche

"Filled with profound wisdom and useful advice, *Wisdom Energy* is a lucid introduction to the key principles and practices of the Buddhism. It demonstrates the authors' remarkable talent for illuminating sometimes complex ideas in a manner that is easily grasped by Westerners. I highly recommend this exceptional book."
—Howard C. Cutler, M.D., co-author of *The Art of Happiness*

160 pages, ISBN 0-86171-170-X, $14.95

Books by the Dalai Lama

IMAGINE ALL THE PEOPLE
A CONVERSATION WITH THE DALAI LAMA ON MONEY, POLITICS, AND LIFE AS IT COULD BE
The Dalai Lama with Fabien Ouaki

The Dalai Lama shares his thoughts on today's issues—money, the economy, the environment, disarmament, and basic human ethics.

192 pages, ISBN 0-86171-150-5, $14.95

THE WORLD OF TIBETAN BUDDHISM
AN OVERVIEW OF ITS PHILOSOPHY AND PRACTICE

"The definitive book on Tibetan Buddhism by the world's ultimate authority."—*The Reader's Review*

"A rare and marvelous opportunity for English-language readers to learn more about [Buddhism and its] spiritual leader…"
—*Library Journal*

224 pages, ISBN 0-86171-097-5, $15.95

THE GOOD HEART
A BUDDHIST PERSPECTIVE ON THE TEACHINGS OF JESUS

His Holiness explores the Gospels, providing a fascinating reading of the Sermon on the Mount, the parable of the mustard seed, the Resurrection, and other selections.

"Sparkling wit and compassionate understanding mark these penetrating insights of the Dalai Lama into spiritual foundations of two of the world's great religious traditions. Highly recommended."
—*Library Journal*

224 pages, ISBN 0-86171-138-6, $14.95

Books by Ayya Khema

"[Ayya Khema is] one of the best Western exponents of the Buddhist path...In disarmingly practical language, she teaches us that true practice is getting the tiny details of life right, the middling moments—thinking before we speak, recognizing greed and generosity in ourselves and others, making the mind pliable at all times."
—Amazon.com

BEING NOBODY, GOING NOWHERE
MEDITATIONS ON THE BUDDHIST PATH

192 pages, ISBN 0-86171-052-5, $14.95

WHO IS MY SELF?
A GUIDE TO BUDDHIST MEDITATION

192 pages, ISBN 0-86171-127-0, $14.95

BE AN ISLAND
THE BUDDHIST PRACTICE OF INNER PEACE

160 pages, ISBN 0-86171-147-5, $14.95

WHEN THE IRON EAGLE FLIES
BUDDHISM FOR THE WEST

224 pages, ISBN 0-86171-169-6, $16.95

To order, call 1-800-272-4050, or visit www.wisdompubs.org

About Wisdom

WISDOM PUBLICATIONS, a not-for-profit publisher, is dedicated to making available authentic Buddhist works by the world's leading Buddhist scholars. We publish our titles with the appreciation of Buddhism as a living philosophy and with the special commitment to preserve and transmit important works from all the major Buddhist traditions.

If you would like more information or a copy of our mail-order catalog, please contact us at:

Wisdom Publications
199 Elm Street,
Somerville, Massachusetts 02144 USA
Telephone: (617) 776-7416 • Fax: (617) 776-7841
Email: info@wisdompubs.org • www.wisdompubs.org

THE WISDOM TRUST

AS A NOT-FOR-PROFIT PUBLISHER, Wisdom Publications is dedicated to the publication of fine Dharma books for the benefit of all sentient beings and dependent upon the kindness and generosity of sponsors in order to do so. If you would like to make a donation to Wisdom, please do so through our Somerville office. If you would like to sponsor the publication of a book, please write or e-mail us for more information.

Thank you.

Wisdom Publications is a non-profit, charitable 501(c)(3) organization and a part of the Foundation for the Preservation of the Mahayana Tradition (FPMT).